The impact of development policies on health

A review of the literature

Diana E. Cooper Weil
Harvard School of Public Health
Boston, MA, USA

Adelaida P. Alicbusan
World Bank, Washington, DC, USA

John F. Wilson
World Bank, Washington, DC, USA

Michael R. Reich
Harvard School of Public Health
Boston, MA, USA

&

David J. Bradley
London School of Hygiene and Tropical Medicine
London, England

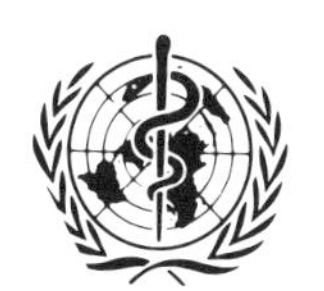

World Health Organization
Geneva
1990

WHO Library Cataloguing in Publication Data

The impact of development policies on health: a review of the literature / Diana E. Cooper Weil . . . [et al.]

1. Economic development 2. Health 3. Public policy 4. Developing countries I. Weil, Diana E. Cooper

ISBN 92 4 156141 6 (NLM Classification: WA 395)

The designations employed and the presentation of the material in this publication do not imply the expression of any opinion whatsoever on the part of the Secretariat of the World Health Organization concerning the legal status of any country, territory, city or area or of its authorities, or concerning the delimitation of its frontiers or boundaries.

The mention of specific companies or of certain manufacturers' products does not imply that they are endorsed or recommended by the World Health Organization in preference to others of a similar nature that are not mentioned. Errors and omissions excepted, the names of proprietary products are distinguished by initial capital letters.

The authors alone are responsible for the views expressed in this publication.

TYPESET IN INDIA
PRINTED IN ENGLAND
90/8478-Macmillan/Clays-5000

Contents

Preface

Generalizations about the relationships between economic development and a population's health status are extremely difficult to make. In many countries economic development has clearly contributed to improving the quality of life and the health status of the population, as measured by indicators such as life expectancy, infant and child mortality, maternal mortality, literacy rates, and access to basic services. It is apparent, however, that economic growth, infrastructure expansion, and agricultural advances do not always coincide with improvements in human well-being. Indeed, there is growing concern that macroeconomic changes may have adverse consequences for poverty alleviation, health, and education. Health authorities are unable, alone, to overcome the resulting health problems.

Three major problems are contributing to a growing "health crisis" which has already increased the burden on the health sector to an insupportable level. Each of these problems has intensified during recent years, indicating the need for policy adjustment. These highly inter-related problems are: the magnitude and diversity of the health hazards associated with development; the cost of treating the diseases caused by industrialization and urbanization; and the need for macroeconomic adjustment, which has resulted in major cuts in the health budgets of many developing countries.

These three daunting problems raise important questions relating to the links between development policy and health status. Although well-planned development policies that incorporate social objectives have contributed to health and quality of life, conditions conducive to ill-health have frequently been created or aggravated by ill-conceived and improperly implemented development schemes. In most cases, the health sector must assume responsibility for the treatment and control of the negative health consequences, which arise largely from circumstances or policies beyond its control.

Over the past decade, the World Health Organization has given prominence to issues of health and development. Following the Conference on Primary Health Care at Alma-Ata in 1978, a programme of Intersectoral Action for Health was initiated in order to promote cooperation between government agencies in different sectors (such as agriculture, education, and health) and to address the health aspects of development policies. In

1986, the technical discussions at the World Health Assembly addressed the issues involved in intersectoral collaboration for health[1] and produced a number of recommendations which formed the basis for Resolution WHA 39.22.

Reflecting these international concerns, WHO and the World Bank began a joint initiative in 1988 on the effects of development policies on health. This initiative had two objectives: first, to review what is known about intersectoral linkages for the prevention of such effects and, secondly, to demonstrate through country studies that health concerns can indeed be taken into account in the design of sectoral development policies. The case studies, it was stressed, would focus on changes in policy that are feasible and implementable.

As an initial step in this collaborative effort, the present publication reviews the literature on the links between development policies and health conditions in five development sectors. While not a critical assessment of the literature, the review does seek to identify major gaps in past and current studies, and to make the case for future ones.

This review, by bringing together the results of diverse studies on the health effects of development policies, seeks to identify the immediate and underlying causes of increases in ill-health in each sector. Each chapter identifies policy components and problems that require further analysis and suggests changes that could help reduce health risks and adverse outcomes. The review provides a basis for future studies that could compare linkages across sectors, assess sectoral connections that heighten health risks, and identify important areas for policy intervention. In addition to serving as a useful document for countries, the review seeks to make key analyses in each development area accessible to policy-makers and analysts in planning authorities, ministries of health, donor agencies, nongovernmental organizations, and international agencies.

Aleya El Bindari Hammad
Adviser on Health and Development Policies,
Office of the Director-General,
World Health Organization,
Geneva, Switzerland

Jeremy J. Warford
Environment Department
World Bank,
Washington, DC, USA

[1] *Intersectoral action for health.* Geneva, World Health Organization, 1986.

Acknowledgements

The authors offer special thanks to the following: Aleya El Bindari Hammad, Adviser on Health and Development Policies, Office of the Director-General, World Health Organization, Geneva, Switzerland; Jeremy J. Warford, Senior Advisor, Environment Department, World Bank, Washington, DC, USA; Bernhard H. Liese, Senior Tropical Diseases Specialist, Population, Health and Nutrition Department, World Bank, Washington, DC, USA; and the members of the WHO Working Group on Intersectoral Action for Health.

In addition, the following people were particularly helpful in the preparation and/or review of portions of this publication: Robert Bos, WHO, Geneva, Switzerland; David Christiani, Harvard School of Public Health, Boston, MA, USA; Greg Goldstein, WHO, Geneva, Switzerland; Pushpa R. J. Herath, WHO, Geneva, Switzerland; James Listorti, World Bank, Washington, DC, USA; Socrates Litsios, WHO, Geneva, Switzerland; Catherine Mulholland, WHO, Geneva, Switzerland; R. Plestina, WHO, Geneva, Switzerland; Alberto Pradilla, WHO, Geneva, Switzerland; Mark Schneider, Pan American Health Organization, Washington, DC, USA; Orville Solon, University of the Philippines, Manila, Philippines.

CHAPTER 1

Introduction

Development policies designed to improve the economic conditions and living standards of communities often have unintended effects on health. While these effects can be positive, many policies create additional health risks for vulnerable groups, thereby compromising the welfare objectives of development policies. Although international agencies and government ministries increasingly recognize these problems, additional efforts need to be made to identify changes in policy that can reduce the health risks arising from development and contribute to health improvement.

Development policies can create or exacerbate the diseases of poverty as well as the health problems of industrialization. Many poor countries now confront this double health burden. Not only must health authorities address the continued prevalence of malnutrition, respiratory infections, diarrhoeal diseases and fevers, and of infections due to viruses, bacteria, and parasites—they also face the emerging problems associated with industrialization and urbanization, including occupational hazards, cardiovascular diseases, cancers, substance abuse, and accidents. The increasing costs of these new problems place additional pressure on the limited national resources available for health service provision and public health activities.

Most development projects now include feasibility studies prior to approval, often with assessments of the environmental impact and occasionally with assessments of the health impact. Some development sectors have made notable progress in this respect. In the field of water resource development, for example, engineers have become more aware of potential environmental and health consequences, and genuine preventive action has become possible on an intersectoral basis.

Numerous obstacles, however, hinder the prediction and measurement of health risks arising from development policies. Planning officials, whether from the health or other sectors, are rarely adequately trained in assessing effects on health. The process of assessment is hampered by poor background data on the population affected, by time restrictions, and by limited financial resources. The tools and methods available for assessment are often inappropriate or too remote from the decision-makers concerned.

Often, even when health consequences are considered, the project modifications required to prevent ill-health may not be undertaken. Sufficient resources may not be available to support the health services needed to treat or control the anticipated health problems. Even with adequate resources, intersectoral cooperation in development planning is difficult to achieve. It is especially difficult to change broad national development strategies and international economic decisions that have negative health consequences.

Some economic policies have severe short-term effects on the welfare of poor populations, even if the long-term effects are calculated to benefit the economy and social welfare as a whole. For this reason, some population groups are especially vulnerable to the adverse effects of development on health; these groups include very poor people, children, women, and some working communities. While certain industrial, agricultural, and energy policies are designed to deal with the immediate health hazards associated with development initiatives, they often fail to provide adequate measures against adverse effects that develop in the long run, especially if those at risk belong to politically marginal groups.

For the purpose of this review, a policy is defined as a broad statement of goals, objectives, and means that creates the framework for government activity (Grindle, 1980). This statement is usually presented as an explicit written document, although a policy can also be implicit or unwritten. In some cases, the absence of an explicit policy may create health hazards. In many cases, failure to implement existing policies contributes to the adverse effects of development activities.

Development policies, for the purposes of this review, are defined as policies designed to encourage economic growth and improve infrastructure, services, industry, commerce, and community development. A broader range of policies also aim to stimulate social and political development. These policies are formulated at the national, regional, and local levels, and may be profoundly affected by international relations, by economic strategies and trends, and by bilateral and international assistance agencies. In addition, the government officials, agencies, and communities involved in making and implementing development policies influence the course and outcome of policies and programmes. The beneficiaries of the policies may not always be those who contribute to, or bear the costs of, their realization.

Development policies and programmes are often thought of as synonymous, but maintaining a distinction between them can be useful from the analytical standpoint. In the implementation process, policies are transformed and modified to become programmes, regulations, guidelines, or the like. This process, too, can have unintended negative consequences for health.

This review considers the impact on health of development policies in five areas outside the health sector, all of which are closely linked to economic growth: (1) macroeconomic policies; (2) agricultural policies; (3) industrial policies; (4) energy policies; and (5) housing policies. The order of the chapters to some extent reflects the importance of each sector to economic growth in developing countries, as well as the potential significance of its impact on health. However, not all policies in each development sector that may adversely affect health are examined. In addition, the review is selective and does not examine policies in certain important areas (such as population, education, and transport). These nevertheless warrant future attention because of their potential effects on health.

In each of the five policy areas, the review of the literature seeks to identify the likely causal associations between policy choice and health outcome, the gaps in knowledge about these associations, and the policy measures that could mitigate negative health effects. Throughout the review, particular attention is given to groups that are especially vulnerable to the adverse effects of development policies. The review also draws attention to disciplinary boundaries that may have restricted previous research on critical intersectoral issues of development. While it does not offer a specific operational framework for action on these issues, it does aim at encouraging new thinking on the subject, as well as providing information for policy discussions and assistance in planning research.

The range of material available and the level of existing knowledge vary greatly between the five policy areas. In some sectors, important reviews of linkages between policy and health are readily available. No attempt is made to repeat this work. Often, however, even detailed reviews of the links between socioeconomic conditions and health have failed to investigate the origins of these conditions in specific sectoral policies. Policy recommendations, if they are offered at all, tend to be general and rarely include an analysis of the likely health costs and benefits.

Readers should bear in mind that this report is subject to the limitations common to reviews of material covering broad areas. It focuses primarily on English-language sources, and, even in the literature in English, important references may have been missed, despite the authors' best efforts to identify relevant documents. The report is also limited in its objectives. No attempt is made to weigh the costs and benefits of development policies in terms of health. The interactive effects of concurrent policies within and between development sectors are not explored. And the report does not analyse problems of country differences and ways in which the impact of development policies might vary according to national responses. Finally, no priorities for policy action in the development sectors are suggested, because of the great variations in health and social conditions across countries.

This review examines how national development policies may create conditions of ill-health for the communities they are intended to benefit, or for those overlooked in development planning. It explores how changes in policy and improvements in implementation can mitigate negative effects and enhance health conditions. The findings suggest that country case studies and other forms of analysis are sorely needed to improve our understanding of how the design and implementation of development policies affect health conditions in developing countries.

Reference

Grindle, M. (1980) Policy content and context in implementation. In: Grindle, M., ed. *Politics and policy implementation in the Third World*. Princeton, Princeton University Press.

CHAPTER 2

Macroeconomic policies

Since the mid-1970s, most developing countries have been increasingly obliged to make adjustments in their economies, in response to macroeconomic problems of imbalance between aggregate demand and supply, inflation, unemployment, and shortage of foreign exchange. The sources of these problems are both external and domestic. Adverse international economic conditions during the greater part of the 1970s and the early 1980s (e.g. oil shocks, world recession, deteriorating terms of trade, debt crises, etc.) have led to many major macroeconomic problems. These have been further compounded by the implementation of domestic policies that discriminate against traditional products and exports (Behrman, 1988).

Thus, in recent years, policies to cope with macroeconomic problems—usually called macroeconomic adjustment or stabilization programmes—have been implemented in several developing countries (Addison & Demery, 1985). They are often carried out in collaboration with the International Monetary Fund, the World Bank, and other international lenders, and the policy packages employed usually have a mixture of objectives. The short-term objectives generally include reductions in balance-of-payments deficits, inflation, and government budgetary deficits; the long-term goals may include the privatization of public enterprises, a shift towards a market-oriented system, or rapid economic growth. Policy measures typically include currency devaluation, reductions in government spending, monetary restrictions, trade liberalization, reform of pricing policies, and wage restraints.

This chapter reviews the available evidence on the impact of macroeconomic policies on the health status of poor people in developing countries. The literature on this subject addresses the relevant issues in terms of macroeconomic policies developed in the context of economic adjustment or stabilization programmes in developing countries. No special meaning is attached to the distinction between adjustment and stabilization programmes in this review. Both types of programme are devised to deal with macroeconomic problems of the nature cited above. Their only difference is that stabilization programmes are intended to tackle short-term problems by effecting reductions in expenditure in order to adjust domestic demand to the reduced level of capital inflows (Davies & Sanders, 1988; World Bank, 1989). Adjustment programmes are designed to deal with the long-term structural causes of problems; as such, they encompass changes in relative prices and reforms of public institutions aimed at making the economy more efficient in the use of productive resources and thereby promoting sustainable growth.

The chapter is in five parts. The first presents the conflicting views of observers on the impact of macroeconomic policies on health status. The next discusses how policies to restructure public expenditure may affect social service provision. Evidence on the role of government expenditure *vis-à-vis* the nutritional status of the poor is discussed in connection with reductions in spending on public health and in food subsidy programmes. The third section highlights the relationship between trade policies and food supply and prices. Also discussed is the impact of the production of crops for export on the cultivation of food crops; and evidence is presented on the nutritional implications of policies to promote the production of export crops. The fourth section focuses on the distributional consequences of economic adjustment policies. Evidence is presented on ways in which adjustment policies may affect rural-urban terms of trade, and the consequences for poverty alleviation are discussed. Evidence is also presented on ways in which households may vary their nutrient intakes in response to changes in income and relative prices. The conclusions are given in the final section, together with the implications for policy design, methods, and research.

The choice of topics is constrained by the scarcity of relevant studies. Unfortunately, most studies in this area have focused on the nutritional impact of economic adjustment policies rather than on health. The consequences on health, if addressed at all, are usually treated theoretically: relatively few studies have attempted to measure or evaluate them. Given this bias in the literature, the evidence assembled in this review often emphasizes the impact of adjustment policies on household nutrition. The intention is not however, to equate nutrition with health. The authors recognize that the undue emphasis on nutritional effects is a serious shortcoming in the literature. This point is taken up further in the concluding section of the chapter.

Conflicting views on the impact of adjustment policies

Adjustment with a human face

Several observers have stressed that recent economic recessions and associated adjustment programmes in developing countries are having a markedly deleterious effect on health and nutrition among the poor of those countries (Jolly, 1985, 1988; Jolly & Cornia, 1984; UNICEF, 1984; Inter-American Development Bank, 1985; World Food Council, 1985). For example, in an analysis of the effects of economic adjustment programmes during the period 1982–84 in several Latin American countries, the Inter-American Development Bank (1985) concluded that "the social cost in terms of reducing living standards, high inflation, and high unemployment has been tremendous and unequally distributed". In another study, Jolly (1988) cited some evidence of rising malnutrition in African countries during the economic decline of the early 1980s. He reported that the proportion of children moderately or severely malnourished almost doubled between 1980 and 1983 in such countries as Botswana, Burundi and Ghana. Smaller increases were recorded for other countries, but base levels were high, e.g., 20% in Lesotho, 30% in Rwanda, and 45% in Madagascar. During the period in question, almost two-thirds of the developing countries recorded negligible or even negative growth in gross domestic product (GDP) per capita—the situation being worst in low-income African countries. Jolly argued that the effect of this decline in average per capita income is magnified in the case of the poor, since recessions result in severe cutbacks in employment and wages. He also cited the tendency for health and other social services to be cut more than other sectors of government spending.

On the basis of the foregoing observations, UNICEF (1984), Jolly & Cornia (1984), and Jolly (1985, 1988) called for special measures to mitigate the impact of adjustment programmes on the poor. Referred to as "adjustment with a human face", these measures are intended primarily to raise the consumption levels of the poor to the basic-needs minimum during the adjustment periods when restraints on consumption levels in general are greatest. Jolly identified three types of policy action for improving the welfare of the poor in this context: first, the goals of the adjustment policy should clearly acknowledge a concern for basic human welfare and be committed to protecting the minimum nutritional levels of the most vulnerable segments of the population. Secondly, the implementation of the adjustment programme should include measures to maintain a minimum floor for nutrition and other basic human needs, depending on what the country can sustain in the long run; measures to restructure the productive sectors in order to enhance the productivity of small producers (via easier access to credit, internal markets, etc.) and promote labour-intensive investments; and measures to solicit international support for these aspects of adjustment, particularly in the form of long-term finance. And, thirdly, a system should be developed for monitoring nutrition levels and the human situation during the adjustment period. Thus adjustment policies should not be concerned only with inflation, balance-of-payments problems, and the growth of the gross national product (GNP)—but also with nutrition and health conditions, food balances, and the development of human resources.

Uncertainty about impact of adjustment programmes

While Jolly and others have maintained that economic adjustment programmes systematically have a magnified adverse effect on health and nutrition in developing countries, others have argued that there is still considerable uncertainty about the overall impact of such programmes on the poor (Behrman, 1988; Preston, 1986). As Behrman suggests, household decisions are the most immediate determinants of health and nutrition, and such decisions are guided by the value of household assets and the price of goods. Since households have a considerable capacity for substitution among products, and even actitivities, in response to changes in economic variables, the impact of recession and adjustment policies on health and nutrition would, on average, be softened rather than magnified. Well-documented examples of the substitution possibilities available to households include: short-run and long-run migration in response to employment options; substitution of less costly sources of nutrients in response to adverse shifts in relative prices or income; and substitution of informal for formal sector activities (Behrman, 1988).

For the very poor, however, substitution possibilities can be severely limited. There are, for example, health risks associated with the substitution of less nutritious food items for more nutritious ones. Forced migration involving either household fragmentation or loss of accommodation is unlikely to be without its cost in health. Some households may lose their flexibility as regards consumption, production, or employment, if they have already made all the substitutions possible for them. And since unemployment involves health risks even in prosperous countries, it would be remarkable if it did not involve them in more marginal situations. Consequently, there can be little uncertainty regarding the impact of adjustment programmes on the households in question. A decline in real income, which an adjustment programme will usually bring about (e.g., through higher commodity prices or reduced public spending for social programmes), can have particularly adverse effects on the health of the very poor.

The linkages between economic outcomes and health and nutritional status are both complex and dynamic in nature. This makes it difficult to formulate precise models and to pin down empirically the overall consequences of adjustment policies on the health status of the poor. In many cases the empirical basis for analysing and monitoring effects on health and nutrition is very weak; and often, deductions are made on the basis of imperfect information (Behrman, 1988). In his review of country case-studies which evaluated the impact of economic adjustment programmes on health and nutrition (e.g., Cornia et al., 1988; UNICEF, 1984), Behrman pointed out that these studies did not explicitly formalize the links between recession and adjustment policies and the deterioration in the health status of children. Instead, they used secondary data to characterize some of the links relating to unemployment, the composition of public expenditure, and major indicators of health and nutrition. In Behrman's view, these studies provide a useful catalogue of trends, but with relatively little direct evidence of a causal linkage between adjustment programmes and deterioration in health status.

Both Jolly and Behrman acknowledge, however, that recessions and adjustment policies could have adverse effects on the health and nutrition of the poor. The differences in their findings are only a matter of degree. While Jolly and others claimed that adjustment policies had a significant deleterious effect on health and nutrition, Behrman suggested that the impact may be only slight. Behrman's conclusion was based on his review of selected studies which analysed the links between adjustment policies and the nutritional status of households, primarily through households' responses to changes in relative prices and income. These studies, as well as those assembled by Cornia et al., are discussed in other sections of this chapter.

Links between economic adjustment policies and health

It is not an easy task to describe in detail the main links between economic adjustment policies and health or the nutritional status of households, since they are numerous and complex. None the less, Addison & Demery (1985) have presented a framework for analysing the effects of economic adjustment policies on income distribution. Pinstrup-Andersen (1987) has provided an outline of the principal relationships between human nutrition and variables affected by economic crises and adjustment programmes. Figure 1 illustrates the major components of the adjustment process and shows how complex they are.

Behrman (1988) considered that no empirical study had so far examined all the links between economic adjustment programmes and health and nutrition in developing countries. However, several studies have systematically examined some of the critical links in the process. Hundreds of macro models in the Keynes–Tinbergen–Klein tradition exist, and these have generally concentrated on estimating the impact of adjustment policies on aggregate output or employment in the context of developing economies (e.g. Lau, 1975; Beltran del Rio & Schwartz, 1986). In recent years, approaches of this kind have relied mainly on social-accounting matrix and computable general-equilibrium models (e.g., Dervis et al., 1983; Pyatt & Thorbecke, 1976; Taylor, 1983). In general, the studies have shown that adjustment policies have a significant impact on macro variables such as employment and aggregate supply, and this is fed back through the distribution of income and relative prices. As Behrman suggested, it is through this feedback mechanism that adjustment policies may potentially alter health and the nutritional well-being of households. Thus, changes in households' real incomes and in the prices of food and other commodities are likely to be reflected in food consumption and nutritional or health status, although probably with a time lag.

One drawback of some of the above-mentioned studies is that, while the models are based on macro variables in the aggregate, the health risks associated with adjustment programmes may be confined largely to the lower end of the income distribution curve. If adjustment policies contribute to higher unemployment and lower output over time, for instance, the health consequences would be more pronounced among the poorest individuals than an aggregate measure for a region or country would suggest. Meanwhile, there have been a number of studies in developed countries covering the health effects of unemployment caused by economic recession (Westcott et al., 1985). These studies show that, where unemployment over extended periods has increased as a result of recession, the associated psychological, economic, and social conditions have led to a broad spectrum of health problems—higher infant mortality rates and increases in mental illness, cardiovascular disease, suicide,

Fig. 1. Schematic overview of principal relationships between human nutrition and variables influenced by economic crises and macroeconomic adjustment policies

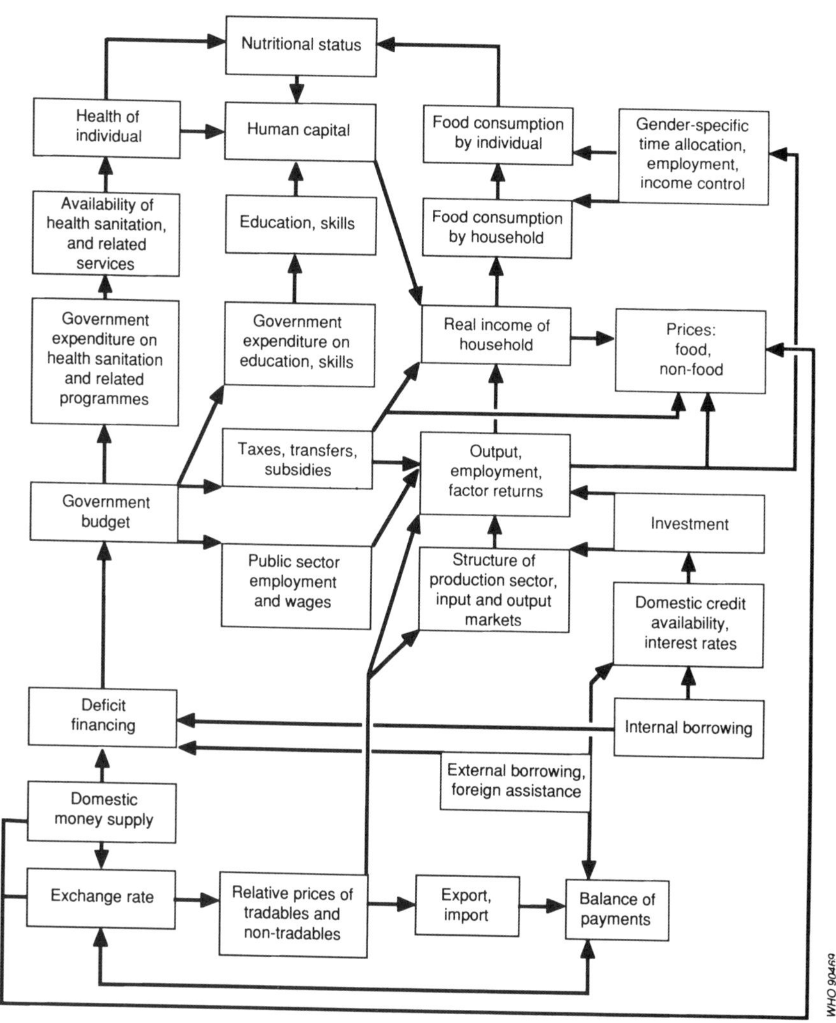

Source: Pinstrup-Andersen, 1987.

alcohol dependence, and drug abuse. The analyses have focused, however, on defining the links between recession, unemployment, and health, and the role of macroeconomic policies in the context of such links is not covered.

Public expenditure and health status

The restructuring of public expenditure as part of economic adjustment programmes may affect health and nutrition, primarily because of the vulnerability of the social sectors to cuts in government spending. This section examines the empirical evidence on this subject, and presents findings from case-studies in different countries on the association between government spending on social services and trends in certain health indicators. It also summarizes the evidence concerning the nutritional impact of food subsidy programmes.

Financing policies for public health are not included in this section, as the subject is too wide. Suffice it to note that several studies done in this area have suggested the need to reconsider financing policies for public health services in developing countries (de Ferranti, 1985; Birdsall, 1985; Jimenez, 1984; Ainsworth, 1984). Health care in these countries has generally been provided free, financed from general taxation. This practice, coupled with an increasing scarcity of fiscal resources, has led to chronic funding problems in the public health sector and contributed to poor-quality services and failure to implement health improvement programmes. The poorest households are usually the ones that suffer most in terms of restricted access to the limited amount of services offered, and that benefit least from the subsidies included in the provision of public health care.

A number of solutions are proposed for these financing problems. One is the institution of pricing reforms in the public health sector, according to different types of health service: preventive services which are not patient-related (e.g., disease control programmes, sanitation, health education) to be provided free; patient-related preventive services (e.g., immunization, maternal and child health care) to be provided at a subsidized cost to users; and curative care (e.g., sale of medicine or drugs, outpatient and inpatient care) to be subject to a charge that reflects the economic cost of providing it. Strengthening the role of the private sector in the supply and financing of health services is another proposed solution. It is argued that the reorientation of health financing policies according to these proposals would improve cost recovery in the public health sector, increase the overall supply of public and private health services, and reduce inequities in the distribution of health resources. It is far from clear how it would affect the very poor, for good or ill, in practice.

Vulnerability of social sectors to cuts in expenditure

The conventional wisdom is that, with increasing budgetary restraints and accompanying shifts in priorities, the social sectors become vulnerable to budgetary cutbacks. However, there are not enough empirical findings to support this assertion, and the available evidence is rather mixed. Thus, from a joint World Health Organization/World Food Programme study (1988) on the health impacts of adjustment programmes in the African region, it appears that, in more than half the cases studied, the health sector has been the first to suffer a cutback when there were budgetary constraints. Reduced health expenditure results in a severe decline in the quality of the health infrastructure, besides limiting supplies of pharmaceuticals.

By contrast, in their study of 37 developing countries for various periods between 1972 and 1980, Hicks & Kubisch (1983, 1984) found that the social sectors were those most protected from cuts in government expenditure, as compared with such sectors as defence, production, and infrastructure (Table 1). They further found that expenditure on the social sectors tended to be more stringently protected in low-income countries than in middle-income countries.

Demery & Addison (1987a) reached similar conclusions for selected countries that had undergone structural adjustments during the early 1980s. In Indonesia, for instance, they found that the Repelita IV Plan entailed shifts in investment priorities in favour of the social sectors at the expense of the productive sectors such as manufacturing, mining, and transport. In Brazil and Chile, aggregate public health expenditure was cut but the commitment of real per capita resources to primary health, nutrition, and basic sanitation—programmes intended to benefit the poor—substantially increased during the adjustment periods. However, in their study of the sub-Saharan African countries, Demery & Addison (1987b) found that, in the 1980s, the restructuring of public expenditure was in general oriented towards agriculture and away from the social sectors. The increasing share allotted to agriculture partly reflected the influence of the World Bank, which had been concerned about protecting budgetary allocations for the improvement of agricultural productivity.

Table 1. Reductions in government expenditure in 37 developing countries, 1972–1980

	Social	Defence/ Administration	Production	Infra-structure	Miscellaneous[a]
Average percentage change in real expenditure	−5	−8	−11	−22	−7
Index of vulnerability[b]	0.4	0.6	1.2	1.7	0.8
Low-income countries ($n=17$)	0.2	0.9	0.6	1.2	0.5
Middle-income countries ($n=20$)	0.5	0.4	1.7	1.9	1.1

[a] Largely transfers to local governments.

[b] Calculated as e_j/E, where e_j is the percentage change in expenditure on the *jth sector, and E* is the percentage change in total expenditure. In this case, $E=-13$.

Adapted from Hicks & Kubisch, 1984. Reproduced by permission of the publisher.

Original data from: International Monetary Fund; *Government finance statistics yearbook, vol. VI. 1982; Government finance statistics,* **37**(7), 1983; and *International financial statistics yearbook.* 1979.

While evidence on the vulnerability of social sectors to budgetary cutbacks is mixed, there is good evidence, from two sets of empirical studies, of the direct impact of social service expenditure on the poor. The first set shows that cuts in such expenditure are related to a decline in health status. The sources are country case studies which have catalogued trends in public expenditure and health indicators over a defined period. Usually the study period was one of economic crisis (e.g., the aftermath of the 1970s oil-price rises, and the world recession of the 1980s) when adjustment policies were in operation. The second set focuses on the effects of food subsidy programmes on nutrition. These programmes are concerned with questions of income distribution and, at times, are implemented to mitigate the adverse effects of economic adjustments on real incomes and the nutritional well-being of the poor. On account of increasing budgetary constraints, an important aspect of food subsidy programmes in developing countries is their cost-effectiveness. Measures of various kinds have been devised to make them as cost-effective as possible, e.g., food supplementation programmes targeted to specific groups such as children and pregnant or lactating women; and food coupons and ration schemes targeted to needy households. The targeting of food subsidies may permit reductions in government expenditure without severe effects on nutrition (Pinstrup-Andersen, 1987).

Government expenditure cuts and health status

Cornia et al. (1988) compiled evidence from case studies showing a direct association between cuts in government expenditure on health and other social services and deterioration in health status. Case studies were presented from ten countries: Botswana, Brazil, Chile, Ghana, Jamaica, Peru, Philippines, the Republic of Korea, Sri Lanka, and Zimbabwe. They showed that the nutritional status of children had deteriorated in all of them, except the Republic of Korea and Zimbabwe. Some of the findings are reviewed below.

In the Philippines, per capita GDP fell by about 3% annually over the period 1979–84. As a result of worsening economic conditions, real per capita public expenditure declined steadily during this period. Per capita public expenditure on health, housing, and other basic social services in 1984 came to only about one-third of the 1979 level (UNICEF, 1988a). A general deterioration in health status was observed, as manifested by higher morbidity, especially from such diseases as diarrhoea, pneumonia, and tuberculosis.

In Ghana, budgetary restraints, coupled with accelerating inflation, made it very difficult to allocate adequate resources to the social sectors, expenditure on which fell from 18% of the GNP in 1972 to 10% in 1982 (UNICEF, 1988b). Since per capita GNP declined by nearly one-third over this period, expenditure on the social sectors had actually fallen sharply in real terms. This resulted in acute shortages of drugs and equipment in the health sector. The decline in health service provision coincided with, and probably contributed to, an increased incidence of such diseases as yaws.

Similarly, in Jamaica, economic stagnation and rapid inflation resulted in sharp declines in public expenditure during the first half of the 1980s. Social expenditure fell by 44% in real terms over the period 1981–85 (Boyd, 1988). In Peru, per capita GDP declined at a rate of about 2% annually over the period 1977–84. Social services accounted for only 18% of total government spending for the period, as compared with 26% in 1968–76 (Figueroa, 1988). In both countries, health conditions deteriorated in terms of reduced health capital stock (e.g., hospitals, clinics, and equipment) or increased incidence of communicable diseases. In Peru, it was estimated that, during the study period, about 44% of children under 6 years of age were malnourished.

By contrast, Zimbabwe experienced an increase in per capita GDP of nearly 2% annually over the period 1980–85. Health expenditure increased only marginally in real terms during this period (Davies & Sanders, 1988). However, the pattern of spending changed, with a rise in the share of the preventive services and a fall in the share of the medical care services. Higher grants were also allocated to organizations providing health care services at the local level in outreach programmes. As a result of this reorientation of health care services, Zimbabwe recorded a notable improvement in health status, especially among children.

Effects of food subsidies on incomes and nutrition

Food subsidies are one form of social expenditure of direct relevance to health and have been studied in some detail for several countries. Pinstrup-Andersen (1985, 1987, 1988) surveyed existing studies on the impact of food subsidies on poor households in terms of real income, food consumption, and nutritional status. The overall implication of his findings is that reductions in budgetary allocations for food programmes may worsen poverty and decrease nutritional well-being.

Specifically, he reaches three major conclusions. First, there is ample empirical evidence that food subsidy programmes in some developing countries have significantly increased the real incomes of the poor. To cite some examples, the subsidized ration schemes which existed in Sri Lanka until 1979 accounted for about 16% of total income in the poorest households in 1978–79 (Gavan & Chandrasekera, 1979). In Pakistan, subsidized food rations during the mid-1970s represented more than 10% of the incomes of the urban poor (Rogers, 1987), whereas in Egypt the corresponding figures were 13% and 17% for the poorest urban and rural households, respectively (Alderman & Braun, 1984). Research on food ration shops in Kerala, India, showed that rations accounted for about one-half of total income in low-income families (George, 1979). On the basis of a number of cases, Pinstrup-Andersen (1988) reported that in general the value of the food subsidies received by low-income households accounted for 15–25% of their total real income.

Second, evidence from case studies suggests that food subsidies have improved food consumption and calorie intake in poor households. Thus, the ration schemes in Sri Lanka increased daily energy consumption by an average of 63 kcal (263 kJ) per capita, and by 115 kcal (481 kJ) per capita among the poorest decile (Gavan & Chandrasekera, 1979). Similarly, in the Philippines a pilot food subsidy programme increased average daily calorie consumption per adult-equivalent unit by 130 kcal (544 kJ) (Garcia & Pinstrup-Andersen, 1986). Ration schemes contributed an increase of 114 and 250 kcal (477 and 1046 kJ) to the daily per capita energy intake of the urban poor in Pakistan (Rogers, 1981) and Bangladesh (Ahmed, 1979), respectively. Subsidized rations in India allowed the poorest consumers to increase their daily energy consumption by up to 18% (George, 1985).

Finally, there is relatively little direct empirical evidence on the effect of food subsidies on nutritional status as measured anthropometrically. None the less, there is evidence suggesting a positive association between children's weight-for-age and food subsidy programmes, notably in case studies in India (Kumar, 1979) and the Philippines (Garcia & Pinstrup-Andersen, 1986).

Anderson et al. (1981) and Beaton & Ghassemi (1979) have reviewed data from more than 200 supplementary feeding projects. Their findings suggest that supplementary feeding programmes have a significant positive effect on birth weight and on child participants. For example, in Guatemala, village women who received a supplement of more than 20 000 kcal (83 MJ) during pregnancy had babies with higher mean birth weights than women receiving lower supplements. Lechtig et al. (1975) reported that the incidence of low birth weight was cut by half in the group receiving high supplements. In India, the birth weights of infants born to women who received daily protein-energy supplements of 700 kcal (2.9 MJ) and 20 g of protein were significantly higher than those of infants born to a nonsupplemented control group (Iyenger, 1967). Studies of infants and children have shown that supplementary feeding programmes are often associated with improved growth, decreased morbidity, or improved cognitive development (Gopaldas et al., 1975; Freeman et al., 1980). A comprehensive list of studies on the nutritional effects of supplementary feeding programmes for mothers and preschool children has been compiled by FAO (1982, 1985). While in general there were serious methodological shortcomings in the evaluation of these effects, the studies consistently show a positive association between programme input and improved nutrition (FAO, 1985).

Clearly, studies of supplementary feeding programmes show some benefits. However, these are usually small, e.g., the increments in birth weight attributed to the programmes are typically in the range of 40–60 g (Pinstrup-Andersen, 1988). A number of reasons are given for this, the primary one being diversion of supplemented foods to non-targeted household members.

Trade policies and food supply

This section deals with food security, with an emphasis on trade interventions for increasing food supply. This emphasis is justified because of the direct association between food availability and household nutrition. The effect of the production of crops for export on the production of food crops and the nutritional status of households is also discussed.

Policies affecting food supply

Food security is defined by the World Bank as the "access by all people at all times to enough food for an active and healthy life" (World Bank, 1986). Many complex factors contribute to food insecurity; however, they can be dealt with basically by increasing the real income of households so that they can afford to acquire enough food. This can be done through measures such as increasing food supply (through production and imports), subsidizing consumer prices (e.g., food subsidy programmes), and targeting income transfers. Measures used by governments to transfer income include public works programmes aimed at doing so through employment (as in South Asia) and cash transfer payments (as in Ethiopia).

Measures of two types can be taken to increase food supply. The first type aims at changing the volume of food trade (e.g., exchange rate controls, export taxes, import tariffs). Through their impact on the volume of food exports or imports, such measures alter the availability and price of food, and hence, affect consumption and domestic production. The second type is designed to increase domestic production (e.g., subsidizing inputs, investing in agricultural infrastructure). Such measures will result in a greater food supply and reduced food prices only in so far as food is not internationally traded. On the other hand, if food is a traded commodity, then such measures generally have no effect on food supply and prices, because additional output is used to expand exports or substitute for food imports (World Bank, 1986). This section is especially concerned with the consequences of measures of the first type.

Most developing countries have pursued trade policies that keep domestic food prices lower than border prices. A common example is the maintenance of overvalued exchange rates. These result in artificially low domestic food prices by creating an effective subsidy for food imports, or by depressing food exports and thus increasing the local food supply. These low food prices may protect urban consumers and also make it possible to have a low-paid labour force. They may also lead to underinvestment in food production. Recently, such trade policies have come under attack on the grounds that in the long run they may inhibit economic growth, worsen poverty, and frustrate efforts to achieve food security (World Bank, 1986). Low prices also adversely affect food producers, with potentially negative health consequences for small farmers.

None the less, policies that keep domestic food prices low are of direct help in improving, at least in the short run, the real income of those households that are net buyers of food. In countries where many of the people facing chronic food insecurity are the rural landless or the urban poor who must buy their food, lower food prices will improve food security. Although empirical findings on the subject are very limited, the available evidence suggests a positive relationship between low food prices and food security.

A World Bank policy study (World Bank, 1986), which analysed data from 29 countries, showed that food security—as measured by the energy content of the national diet—increases as the price of food decreases when income is held constant. Binswanger & Quizon (1984) analysed the effects of alternative trade policies on chronic food insecurity using an agricultural sector model for India. They found that a simulated increase of wheat imports equal to 10% of the existing supply in the 1970s would have decreased the domestic price of wheat by 15%, that of rice by 6%, and that of coarse grains by 5%. Consequently, real income and cereal consumption for the lowest quartile of the urban population would have risen by about 5%. Similarly, the effects on income and consumption in the lowest quartile of the rural population would have been positive, although to a lesser extent. Binswanger & Quizon concluded that, in India, trade measures leading to lower food prices would reduce chronic food insecurity for the most vulnerable segments of the population.

At this point, an important question to ask is whether trade measures affecting food supply are cost-effective in improving food security. The answer of course depends on how far the measures actually touch the intended beneficiaries, the effect a price change would have on the net incomes of the poor, and the extent to which price distortions in production affect efficiency (World Bank, 1986). Clearly, an examination of the trade-offs involved is needed. For example, policies to maintain overvalued exchange rates can cause a misallocation of resources throughout the economy, with all tradable goods underpriced relative to non-tradable goods. While overvalued exchange rates can hold food prices down, if food products are tradable goods, they can also have a substantial effect on the prices of all agricultural products. In the long run, this may have serious consequences for growth in the agricultural sector, with adverse effects on the demand for labour and wages, i.e., on an important source of income for the poor. Devaluation in the interests of efficiency can result in drastic increases in food prices, and for the poor, modifications in food consumption can mean going hungry: poor households spend at least 55% of their income on food (Pinstrup-Andersen, 1987). However, devaluation, by shifting the rural-urban terms of trade in favour of agriculture, offers the long-term prospect of higher employment and output (Timmer et al., 1983). This is a good reason for considering compensatory measures to soften the adverse short-term effects of a devaluation policy on the poor (e.g., food subsidy programmes, temporary subsidies for food imports). It thus appears that measures to enhance food security should be preceded by a balanced empirical analysis of the effects of changes in food prices in the country concerned.

Export crops versus food crops

Strategies to promote exports are a major component of trade liberalization policies in the adjustment programmes of developing countries. These strategies may consist of direct interventions such as adjustments in export taxes and prices, or indirect interventions such as the simplification of export procedures through the removal of export bans and quotas, the provision of export insurance and credit schemes which may be targeted to certain crops, and priority access to foreign exchange for purchases of imported productive inputs.

The promotion of export crops and its likely impact on the food supply are of particular relevance to household consumption and nutrition. The basic premise is that the increased production of export crops may adversely affect the production of food crops, especially the staples, through competition for productive resources. Relatively little research, however, has been done on this subject, and the available evidence appears not to support the above premise.

Braun & Kennedy (1986) have studied the relationship between cash cropping (involving the production of crops for both domestic and export markets) and the production of food crops (see Fig. 2, which shows some of the linkages between cash crop production and nutritional status investigated by the authors in question). In their analysis of 11 countries, they found that a rapid expansion in cash crop production does not limit staple food production. In fact, countries where the per capita production of basic staples is growing appreciably (e.g., Indonesia, Philippines, and Rwanda) have simultaneously expanded the areas they allocate to cash crops. In Bangladesh, Mali, Nigeria, Peru, and Senegal there is still a positive relationship between the two types of production: where per capita food production is constant or declining, the area allocated to cash crops is likewise constant or declining. Brazil, Guatemala and Kenya provide the only examples of a negative association between increased production of cash crops and per capita food production.

Similar studies have demonstrated that competition between food crops and cash crops is limited and, in some exceptional cases, they are even complementary. In the United Republic of Tanzania, Bryceson (1988) found that cash cropping by peasant households has largely replaced surplus production during normal years; it appeared that, as long as food could be bought in bad years, cash cropping would not undermine household food supplies. Whitehead (1988) reported a positive correlation between food crop production and cash crop production among households in northern Ghana—families either produce enough food crops for their own consumption and cash crops for the market, or not enough food crops and no cash crops. Sharpley (1988) showed that in Kenya, food crops for domestic consumption used up more foreign exchange than export crops did. She concluded that a strong export crop sector would be important for generating foreign exchange that could be used in expanding food production. Longhurst (1988) suggested that certain

Fig. 2. Some linkages between cash crop production and nutritional status at household and intrahousehold level

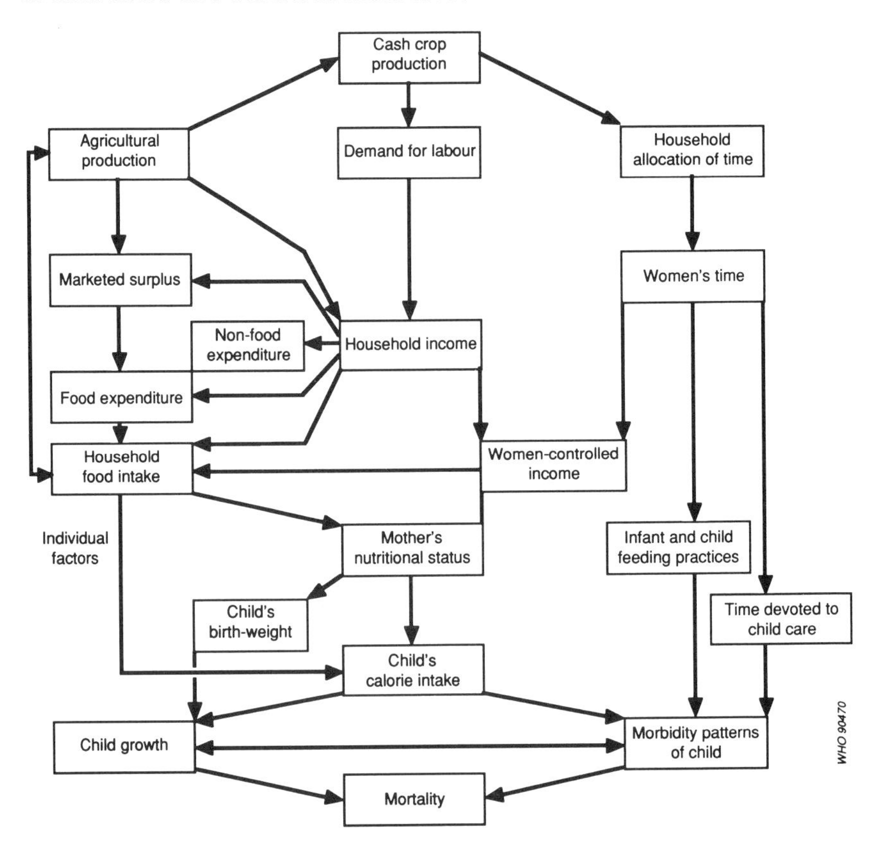

Source: Braun & Kennedy, 1986.

cash crops may be beneficial to food security—specifically in cases where the cash crop is also a food crop, grown by women and easy to process. An example cited is that of groundnuts in Gambia. These contribute 21% of the total calorie intake and 24% of the total protein intake of households during the post-harvest season (International African Institute, 1982); in addition, they provide employment for the women who extract the oil, making them better off and thus perhaps improving child nutrition indirectly. Longhurst further suggested that cash cropping may have negative effects on nutrition when a shift to cash crop production creates uncertainty in household budgets, e.g., in the case of long-maturing tree crops yielding "lumpy" financial returns that all come at one time of the year.

Other observers have also maintained that an increase in export crop production need not result in a lower food supply in the exporting country (Demery & Addison, 1987b; Kirkpatrick & Diakosavvas, 1985). This would depend on two key issues: whether the additional foreign exchange from export crops is sufficient to allow for compensatory food imports; and whether the import of food has priority in the sectoral allocation of foreign exchange. In many developing countries, food imports are more a political issue than an economic consideration. Since food availability and low food prices are of importance in maintaining political stability, there is a strong incentive for governments to use foreign exchange generated by exports to pay for more food imports.

In their study of 30 African countries over the period 1965–83, Kirkpatrick & Diakosavvas (1985) found that cereal imports were generally unaffected by variations in domestic food production. Shortfalls in output were not fully compensated for by food imports, so that food supplies could not be maintained at desired levels. In all but three of the countries studied, the problem was a shortage of foreign exchange due to poor performance in the agricultural export sector. This finding has important implications: it demonstrates the importance of increasing the output potential of agriculture as a whole to ensure a country's ability to maintain its food supply. Simply increasing domestic food production at the expense of export production does not guarantee secured supplies of food (Demery & Addison, 1987b). The optimal mix of food crops and export crops should be dictated by the underlying costs in resources and the comparative advantages involved.

The nutritional consequences of export crop production

Braun & Kennedy (1986) conducted a comprehensive review of the relationship between cash cropping and the nutritional status of households. Their main findings are twofold: first, studies of the effects of cash crop production on income and nutrition have yielded mixed results. Thus Rabeneck (1982), Fleuret & Fleuret (1983), and Harvey & Heywood (1983) found that cash cropping had a positive effect on nutritional status; others have found the opposite (e.g., Dewey, 1979; Hernandez et al., 1974). The same crop appears to be associated with positive nutritional effects in some countries and negative effects in others (Rabeneck, 1982; Hitchings, 1982; Lambert, 1978). Braun & Kennedy suggest that these conflicting results probably reflect the heterogeneity of the situations, as well as differences in the methodological approaches employed.

Secondly, it is usually assumed that a switch from semi-subsistence to commercial agriculture will enhance the ability of households to acquire food, since it will increase family income. There is, in fact, some evidence that cash crop production can result in significant gains in household income. For instance, Kennedy & Cogill (1985) found that, in Kenya, the cash incomes of farmers participating in the sugar outgrowers' scheme were almost double those of non-participants. In contrast, however, Pinstrup-Andersen (1983) has described various situations in which export crop production could negatively affect income. For example, farm-gate prices of export crops could be lower than expected owing to unforeseen export taxes, falling world market prices, and the exploitation of local monopsony (sole buyer) power.

A more important issue, however, is whether the additional household income from cash crops is translated into better nutrition. Here again, the empirical evidence is mixed. Studies among low-income households in Colombia and Nicaragua have shown weak but positive links between income and calorie consumption (Braun & Kennedy, 1986). A study in Nicaragua on the effects of technological innovations on nutrition showed that a 10% increase in household income increased calorie consumption by about 5–6% (IFPRI, 1985). In Colombia, the introduction of high-yielding varieties of maize significantly increased the income of participating households; however, their marginal propensity to spend on calories out of additional income was only 0.1 (Goldman & Overholt, 1981). Hernandez et al. (1974) investigated the effects of cash crop production in a poor village in Mexico. They found that there was no significant decrease in malnutrition among preschool children as measured by weight for age, between 1958 (prior to the introduction of cash crops) and 1971 (13 years after the programme had been implemented). They concluded that the economic gains from cash cropping did not translate into improved nutrition. In the southern highlands of the United Republic of Tanzania, a study by Jakobsen (1978) showed a negative relationship between economic growth in monetary terms and children's growth. Other studies (Rabeneck, 1982; Fleuret & Fleuret, 1983; Harvey & Heywood, 1983), however, have indicated a positive association between cash crop production and income and preschool children's growth.

Why then this discrepancy? Braun & Kennedy (1986) suggest that it may be due to two factors: differences in the indicators used in evaluating outcomes (household food expenditure, family calorie and nutrient consumption, growth, and morbidity), and the question of who controls what kind of income. In many cultures, men handle cash income, and women food income. In a review of projects introducing technological change into rural areas, Tinker (1979) found that the general trend was for nutritional levels to fall as income from cash cropping increased. She concluded that the primary reason for this paradox was the fact that the income from cash crops belonged to men, who then used it for house improvement, giving "prestige" feasts, etc. Similar findings were reported by Katona-Apte (1983) in an analysis of the impact of agricultural projects on nutrition. Agricultural projects can have positive effects on nutrition only where women participate in farm production, as the source of labour, and thus have control over the generation of income. In societies where women hardly contribute towards the family income, cash cropping may not lead to improved nutrition.

Economic adjustment programmes and income distribution

Adjustment programmes in developing countries have paid special attention to restoring incentives for agricultural production, largely through higher prices for producers, devaluation, and reduced control of markets. This reflects efforts by governments to accelerate growth and raise productivity in agriculture, by influencing the adjustment process towards the production of tradable goods. Such a policy may also considerably alter the distribution of income. This section presents evidence on: the effects of economic adjustment programmes on income distribution and the implications for poverty alleviation; and the responsiveness of households to changes in relative prices and income in terms of adjustments in their expenditure on food and their nutrient intake.

The effects of devaluation on income distribution

In their survey of the literature on macroeconomic stabilization policies in developing countries, Addison & Demery (1985) concluded that very little research had been done on the relationship between income distribution and stabilization in those countries. Most studies were inconclusive about the effects of stabilization policies on income distribution. Although some observers have maintained that particular forms of stabilization worsen income distribution (Dervis et al., 1983), on the whole this issue remains an open question. This underlines the need for in-depth case studies in which empirical evidence can be systematically compiled and analysed.

A case in point is that of the impact of exchange rate adjustments on income distribution. Devaluation is a key component of stabilization programmes supported by the International Monetary Fund. It may affect the distribution of income through changes in the relative prices of traded and nontraded goods and changes in real income. But devaluation also interacts with several macro variables like trade (im)balances, (un)employment, and inflation. Given the complex linkages involved, the overall impact of devaluation on income distribution is difficult to nail down empirically.

No generalization can therefore be made regarding this issue. As Addison & Demery (1985) pointed out, whether devaluation actually leads to greater or lesser inequalities of income depends on the specific characteristics of the country in question. Thus, devaluation may improve income distribution if export crops are largely produced by small farmers; it may contribute to inequalities of income if the production of import substitutes is relatively capital-intensive. Similarly, if an export commodity is also the staple food (e.g., rice in Thailand), then devaluation may result in a substantial fall in the real income of the poor.

The foregoing argument is borne out by empirical evidence from case studies. Johnson & Salop (1980) assessed the impact on income distribution of a sustained reduction, achieved through devaluation, in the ratio of prices of nontraded goods to those of traded goods. The analysis was based on case studies of stabilization programmes in four countries: Bolivia (1972–73), Ghana (1966–70), Indonesia (1966–74), and the Philippines (1970–76). They concluded that the impact on income distribution differs according to the underlying structure of the economy. Thus, in Ghana, since the export sector was primarily agricultural, with small producers in the majority, and was an important source of employment for a large segment of the population, effects of a decline in the price ratio on income distribution tended to be of a fairly egalitarian nature.

In the other countries, however, devaluation tended to intensify inequalities of income, especially in the rural areas. In Bolivia, the export sector was made up largely of mineral products, with production concentrated among public enterprises. Agricultural products and simple manufactures represented the nontrade sector, which was dominated by small producers. In the Philippines, the agricultural sector was split between large farms producing export crops and numerous small farms producing staple foods. In Indonesia, the export sector was dominated by petroleum and agricultural products, while the agricultural sector, which employed about two-thirds of the labour force, consisted of public estates planted with export crops and small farms specializing in food crops.

Hence, a decline in the price ratio would tend to shift real income away from agricultural producers in general (in Bolivia), away from small farmers engaged primarily in the production of food crops (in Indonesia and the Philippines), and away from wage-earners employed in the nontrade sector. The beneficiaries would be the urban sector and producers of export goods.

However, Johnson & Salop stress that the overall distributional implications of devaluation are difficult to assess empirically. In Indonesia, for example, the relatively rapid economic growth that took place in the urban sector during the study period had led to increased migration to urban areas. Owing to complications of this nature, the overall impact of devaluation on income distribution becomes far from clear-cut.

The effects of agricultural prices on rural–urban terms of trade

Another measure commonly used to encourage agricultural production is to increase agricultural prices directly. The impact of higher prices for producers on the regional distribution of income has been studied in a few countries. In Côte d'Ivoire, for instance, adjustment policies aimed at increasing agricultural producer prices in line with world prices resulted in improved rural-urban terms of trade and reduced income inequalities to the benefit of rural households (Demery & Addison, 1987a). During the adjustment period of 1980–84, per capita disposable income in urban areas declined by about 11% a year while income in rural areas was reduced by only 1.2%. The ratio of urban to rural income declined to 2:1 in 1985, compared with 3.5:1 in 1980. Stabilization policies in Ghana and the United Republic of Tanzania produced similar results.

Although rural–urban income differentials may have declined as a result of adjustment programmes, it is not clear whether rural poverty has thus been alleviated. At least three considerations are in order here: first, marginal farmers who are net consumers, as opposed to those who are surplus producers, may have been affected adversely by higher producer prices. A good example is provided by Thailand, where about 25% of rice farmers actually consume more rice than they produce (Trairatvorakul, 1984). The income gains from higher rice prices have accrued mainly to large paddy farmers who account for a disproportionately large share of the marketed output. Secondly, in most developing countries, such as the African countries mentioned above, the poorest farm households are engaged primarily in subsistence farming. The benefits of adjustment programmes may be negligible for them unless they can diversify production to include cash crops (Demery & Addison, 1987a). And thirdly, evidence suggests that the higher employment rates associated with higher producer prices and output may not do as much as anticipated to alleviate poverty among the rural landless. Additional employment does not seem to increase the income of agricultural labourers sufficiently to compensate them for their losses as consumers (Ahmed, 1979; Clay, 1981).

Other observers have argued that adjustment programmes have a greater adverse impact on urban poverty than on rural poverty. Pinstrup-Andersen (1985) summarized evidence from developing countries showing that the urban poor suffer most as a result of increases in agricultural prices. Jamal (1985) came to the same conclusion in his study of the adjustment programmes in Uganda. It therefore appears that the overall effect of adjustment programmes in alleviating poverty is questionable. At best, they may only change the composition of poverty without actually reducing it.

Households' responses to changes in income and prices

Several studies have been conducted to estimate the responsiveness of households to changes in prices and incomes. Such responsiveness is often measured in terms of changes in the amount of food bought, expenditure on food, and calorie consumption. Estimates are generally based on cross-sectional data differentiating income groups. These studies provide two important observations: first, since poorer households spend a much larger share of their budgets on food—typically 60–80% (Pinstrup-Andersen, 1987)—than better-off households, they are more responsive to changes in prices and income. In his review of studies covering 11 countries, Alderman (1986) found that the price elasticity of the demand for rice among the poorest 10% of a population was about 80% higher than the mean value for the whole population. Similarly, Pinstrup-Andersen (1985) compiled evidence from studies in eight countries on the price elasticity of the demand for rice among low and high-income population groups. He found that, consistently from country to country, low-income households had more marked responses to changes in rice prices. Elasticity estimates for low-income households vary by country from −0.43 to −4.31, whereas those for high-income groups vary from −0.19 to −1.15. Mellor (1975) estimated that, for every 10% increase in food-grain prices, the poorest households in India would decrease their real expenditure on food grains and on milk products by about 6% and by 18%, respectively.

The corresponding reductions among high-income groups were 0.2% and 1.3%, respectively.

Secondly, large changes in food expenditure, particularly among the poor, do not necessarily imply large changes in nutrient intake. Using aggregate data from 30 countries, Behrman & Deolalikar (1986) found that, for every 10% decline in income, households reduced their average food expendtiture by 8%, while their calorie intake decreased by only 3%. This finding is consistent with the relatively low responses in terms of nutrient intake reported in other studies (e.g., Alderman, 1986; Behrman & Wolfe, 1984; Levinson, 1974; Pitt & Rosenzweig, 1983). As pointed out by Behrman (1988), households may substantially alter the composition of their diet in response to changes in relative prices or income. A decline in income may reduce expenditure on household food, but mainly through a shift to less costly sources of nutrients rather than a reduction in nutrient intake. Behrman argues that if it is true that, in terms of nutrient intake, poor households have a limited response to income changes, as the above studies suggest, "then the impact of economic adjustment policies on nutrients consumed by the poor probably is much less than often assumed" (Behrman, 1988). However, this argument depends largely on precisely who are considered to be "the poor".

Conclusion

On the whole, this review of the literature shows that health and nutrition in developing countries can be adversely affected by economic adjustment programmes. Of course, some of the evidence presented in this review is rather inconclusive; in other instances, the amount of evidence available is limited in the absence of appropriate empirical work. Nevertheless, it seems that, in general, adjustment policies can have a negative effect on the nutritional well-being of the poor in developing countries. This is because adjustment programmes frequently include changes of particular concern to the poor: reductions in real wages, increases in food prices, and cuts in government expenditure on social services (Pinstrup-Andersen, 1987).

The inconclusiveness of the literature on the impact of adjustment programmes has to do with the fact that in many respects—economic, political, etc.—countries are extremely heterogeneous. Hence, experience with adjustment programmes varies substantially from country to country. Undoubtedly, some countries have countered the adverse effects of adjustment programmes better than others. Wherever political commitment to improve the welfare of the poor is strong enough, there is probably a great deal to be learnt from their experience.

Several policy options are open to governments seeking to soften the adverse impacts of adjustment programmes on the poor—for example, a food subsidy programme designed to be cost-effective by being targeted strictly to the vulnerable segments of the population. Experience with food subsidies in Sri Lanka, for example, has important lessons to offer. Another option is to restructure public health expenditure, giving priority to the expansion of primary health care, basic nutrition programmes, basic sanitation services, and other programmes that benefit the poor in particular. Here, there are valuable lessons to be learnt from the experiences of Brazil, Chile, and Zimbabwe. Meanwhile, other options are: to improve employment opportunities for the poor through labour-intensive investment; to ensure access by the poor to educational services; and to increase their access to productive assets by making institutional credit available and through land reform programmes. As Demery & Addison (1987a) have pointed out, policies of this kind will allow the poor to participate in the adjustment process and can help alleviate poverty in the long run.

A wide gap exists between the formulation of policies intended to provide long-term solutions to macroeconomic problems and the implementation of measures to evaluate or monitor the health consequences of policies for the poor. Policy-makers may believe that economic growth at the macro level, which adjustment programmes are intended to bring about, will automatically lead to substantial "trickle-down effects" favouring household nutrition and the alleviation of poverty. This may be why, in formulating policies, they have usually disregarded mechanisms for assessing the distributional and nutritional effects of the adjustments made, let alone for designing auxiliary policies to protect the interests of the poor while remaining consistent with the goals of the adjustment programme (Montes, 1987). Such programmes are not meant to impose a heavy burden on the poor. However, experience in many developing countries suggests that, in the short-term, high inflation, unemployment, and reduced real incomes often result in a redistribution of income that is biased against the poor. This in turn can have serious consequences for nutrition and health.

In a review of its position on structural adjustment policies, it was concluded that the World Bank has yet to develop a set of policies that effectively address the twin objectives of growth and poverty alleviation (Reutlinger, 1987). While the Bank has strongly endorsed growth as the ultimate solution to adjustment difficulties, historically the objective of poverty alleviation has been dealt with through selected projects in the areas of population, health, nutrition, and education, and schemes to provide small farmers with remunerative employment. More recently, an improved approach has been adopted whereby adjustment programmes include specific distributional objectives. A good example is the Agricultural Incentive Programme Credit for Guinea-Bissau proposed in 1986. This is intended to support policies aimed at raising official producer prices, in order to encourage the production of food and export crops. Since food prices for consumers will also be increased, the adjustment operations allow for the use of food-aid funds as a buffer for those who will be adversely affected by the increases. Specifically, the proceeds from government food-aid sales are intended to go towards increasing the wages of low-income urban households in order to compensate them for a decline in real income due to the higher food prices. The adjustment programme also includes arrangements for monitoring the effects of such prices on urban and rural food consumption as well as on crop production. Similar adjustment programmes with special emphasis on poverty alleviation are currently being considered in Mauritania and Morocco.

Partly because the links between macroeconomic policies and health are numerous and complex, the literature is inconclusive. The various policy instruments that go to make up an economic adjustment programme can have conflicting effects, thus making it difficult to be precise about the overall effect of the programme. Major gaps also exist in empirical evidence of the effects of adjustment programmes on health. The limited studies done in this area so far indicate the specific adjustment policies that may especially affect social welfare, the distribution of income, and household nutrition. These policies include currency devaluation, measures to promote exports, pricing reforms and subsidies, labour and wage policies, and provisions concerning public expenditure and social services. But not a single study has examined all the major links between economic adjustment programmes and health and nutrition. Different sets of related studies have therefore been used in this review in an attempt to piece together the scattered evidence available on the various processes involved in the linkage between adjustment policies and health conditions. The effects of these policies are still evaluated almost exclusively in terms of changes in nutritional status, without any reference to their implications for health. In general, the studies do not provide any formal or explicit interpretation of the effects on nutrition in terms of the changes that are likely to occur in health status. More research is needed for a better understanding of the intricate links between adjustment programmes and the responses of households to changes in macroeconomic conditions, particularly as they affect health in developing countries.

In a detailed discussion of research needs in this area, Pinstrup-Andersen (1987) suggested that a number of in-depth country studies should be undertaken (Addison & Demery (1985), among others, share this view). These studies should seek: to improve knowledge of the processes whereby specific adjustment policies may affect the nutritional status of the poor; to establish a basis for redesigning adjustment programmes to combine efficiency with equity; and to provide generally applicable examples that can be used in predicting the probable consequences of economic adjustments and in policy-making. The economic structure of each country should be closely examined, as there are wide national variations, and it should be remembered both that the poor are a highly varied group and that adjustment policies and their effects are not instantaneous. Appropriate allowances should be made for time lags, and analyses should cover several years. The poor should be grouped according to age and gender, as well as by occupation (e.g., landless agricultural workers, semi-subsistence farmers, non-farm labourers, and persons self-employed in the informal sector (examples of this will be found in Sahn, 1983; Trairatvorakul, 1984; Garcia & Pinstrup-Andersen, 1986).

Several analytical approaches may be considered for evaluating the links between adjustment policies and nutritional and health status: comparative analysis, partial equilibrium econometric analysis, and the use of computer-generated equilibrium models, input-output models, or social accounting matrices. Pinstrup-Andersen (1987) discussed the merits and weaknesses associated with each approach, concluding that the final choice would depend on the objectives of the study, the availability of data and the relative costs. He none the less suggested that, in many cases, a comparative approach based on data from several years, together with partial equilibrium econometric analysis, would be the most appropriate one. The specifications of the econometric models, of course, may vary according to circumstances in the countries under study.

References

Addison, T. & Demery, L. (1985) *Macro-economic stabilization, income distribution and poverty: a preliminary survey*. London, Overseas Development Institute.

Ahmed, R. (1979) *Foodgrain supply, distribution, and consumption policies within a dual pricing mechanism: a case study of Bangladesh*. Washington, DC, International Food Policy Research Institute (Research Report 8).

Ainsworth, M. (1984) *User charges for social sector finance: policy and practice in developing countries*. Washington, DC, World Bank, (CPD Discussion Paper No. 1984–6).

Alderman, H. (1986) *The effect of food price and income changes on the acquisition of food by low-income households*. Washington, DC, International Food Policy Research Institute.

Alderman, H. & Braun, J. von (1984) *The effects of the Egyptian food ration and subsidy system on income distribution and welfare*. Washington, DC, International Food Policy Research Institute (Research Report 45).

Anderson, M. A. et al. (1981) *Nutrition intervention in developing countries. Study I: Supplementary feeding*. Cambridge, MA, Oelgeschlager, Gunn & Hain.

Beaton, G. H. & Ghassemi, H. (1979). *Supplementary feeding programmes for young children in developing countries*. New York, United Nations Children's Fund.

Behrman, J. R. (1988) The impact of economic adjustment programs. In: Bell, D. E. & Reich, M. R., ed. *Health, nutrition, and economic crises: approaches to policy in the Third World*. Dover, MA, Auburn House Publishing Co.

Behrman, J. R. & Deolalikar, A. (1986) *Is variety the spice of life? Implications for nutrient responses to development*. Philadelphia, University of Pennsylvania (mimeographed document).

Behrman, J. R. & Wolfe, B. L. (1984) More evidence on nutrition demand: income seems overrated and women's schooling underemphasized. *Journal of development economics*, 14(1–2): 105–128.

Beltran del Rio, A. & Schwartz, R. (1986) *Bibliography of Latin American macroeconomic models*. Philadelphia, Wharton Econometric Forecasting Associates (mimeographed document).

Binswanger, H. & Quizon, J. (1984) *Distributional consequences of alternative food policies in India*. Washington, DC, World Bank (Report No. ARU 29).

Birdsall, N. (1985) *Cost recovery in health and education: bank policy and operations*. Washington, DC, Population, Health and Nutrition Department, World Bank.

Boyd, D. (1988) The impact of adjustment policies on vulnerable groups: the case of Jamaica, 1973–1985. In: Cornia, G. A. et al., ed., *Adjustment with a human face. Vol. 2. Country case studies*. Oxford, Clarendon Press pp. 126–155.

Braun, J. von & Kennedy, E. (1986) *Commercialization of subsistence agriculture: income and nutritional effects in developing countries*. Washington, DC, International Food Policy Research Institute.

Bryceson, D. F. (1988) Peasant cash cropping vs. food self-sufficiency in Tanzania: a historical perspective. *Institute of Development Studies bulletin*, 19(2): 37–46.

Clay, E. J. (1981) Poverty, food insecurity, and public policy in Bangladesh.

Food policy issues in low-income countries. Washington, DC, World Bank (Staff Working Paper No. 473), pp. 48–84.

Cornia, G. A. et al., ed. (1987/1988) *Adjustment with a human face. Vol. 1. Protecting the vulnerable and promoting growth; Vol. 2. Country case studies*. Oxford, Clarendon Press.

Davies, R. & Sanders, D. (1988) Adjustment policies and the welfare of children: Zimbabwe, 1980–1985. In: Cornia, G. A. et al., ed. *Adjustment with a human face. Vol. 2. Country case studies*. Oxford, Clarendon Press, pp. 272–299.

de Ferranti, D. (1985) *Paying for health services in developing countries: an overview*. Washington, DC, World Bank (Staff Working Paper No. 721).

Demery, L. & Addison, T. (1987a) *The alleviation of poverty under structural adjustment*. Washington, DC, World Bank.

Demery, L. & Addison, T. (1987b) Food insecurity and adjustment policies in sub-Saharan Africa: a review of the evidence. *Development policy review*, 5(2): 177–198.

Dervis, K. et al. (1983) *General equilibrium models for development policy*. Cambridge, Cambridge University Press.

Dewey, K. (1979) Commentary—agricultural development, diet and nutrition. *Ecology of food and nutrition*, **8**: 265–273.

FAO (1982) *Evaluation of nutrition interventions*. Rome, Food and Agriculture Organization of the United Nations (FAO Food and Nutrition Paper 24).

FAO (1985) *Nutritional implications of food aid: an annotated bibliography*. Rome, Food and Agriculture Organization of the United Nations (FAO Food and Nutrition Paper 33).

Figueroa, L. (1988) Economic adjustment and development in Peru: towards an alternative policy. In: Cornia, G. A. et al., ed. *Adjustment with a human face. Vol. 2. Country case studies*. Oxford, Clarendon Press, pp. 156–183.

Fleuret, P. & Fleuret, A. (1983) Socio-economic determinants of child nutrition in Taita, Kenya: a call for discussion. *Culture and agriculture*, **19**: 8–20.

Freeman, H. E. et al. (1980) Nutrition and cognitive development among rural Guatemalan children. *American journal of public health*, **70**: 1277–1285.

Garcia, M. & Pinstrup-Andersen, P. (1986) *Pilot food subsidy scheme in the Philippines: impact on income, food consumption, and nutritional status*. Washington, DC, International Food Policy Research Institute.

Gavan, J. & Chandrasekera, I. S. (1979) *The impact of public foodgrain distribution on food consumption and welfare in Sri Lanka*. Washington, DC, International Food Policy Research Institute (Research Report 13).

George, P. S. (1979) *Public distribution of foodgrains in Kerala: income distribution implications and effectiveness*. Washington, DC, International Food Policy Research Institute (Research Report 7).

George, P. S. (1985) *Some aspects of procurement and distribution of foodgrains in India, food subsidies*. Washington, DC, International Food Policy Research Institute (Working Paper No. 1).

Goldman, R. & Overholt, C. (1981) *Nutrition intervention in developing countries. Study VI. Agricultural production, technical change and nutritional goals*. Cambridge, MA, Oelgeschlager, Gunn and Hain.

Gopaldas, T. et al. (1975) *Project poshak, vol. 1*. New Delhi, CARE.

Harvey, P. & Heywood, P. (1983) *Nutrition and growth in Simbu, vol. 4*. Papua New Guinea, Simbu Provincial Government, Office of Environment and Conservation.

Hernandez, M. et al. (1974) Effect of economic growth on nutrition in a typical community. *Ecology of food and nutrition*, **4**: 283–291.

Hicks, N. & Kubisch, A. (1983) *The effects of expenditure reductions in developing countries*. Washington, DC, World Bank (mimeographed documents).

Hicks, N. & Kubisch, A. (1984) Cutting government expenditures in LDCs. *Finance and development*, **21**: 37–39.

Hitchings, J. (1982) *Agricultural determinants of nutritional status among Kenyan children with model of anthropometric and growth indicators*. Ph.D. dissertation, Stanford University.

IFPRI (1985) *Nutritional effects of technological change in agriculture and related public policies and projects: selected case studies*. Final report submitted by the International Food Policy Research Institute to the International Fund for Agricultural Development, Washington, DC (mimeographed document).

Inter-American Development Bank (1985) *Economic and social progress in Latin America: external debt-crisis and adjustment*. Washington, DC.

International African Institute (1982) *Village food systems in West Africa*. London (mimeographed document).

Iyenger, L. (1967) Effect of dietary supplementation late in pregnancy on the expectant mother and her newborn. *Indian journal of medical research*, **55**: 85–89.

Jakobsen, O. (1978) *Economic and geographical factors influencing child malnutrition: a study from the southern highlands, Tanzania*. United Republic of Tanzania, University of Dar es Salaam (Research paper 52).

Jamal, V. (1985) *Structural adjustment and food security in Uganda*. Geneva, International Labour Office (ILO World Employment Programme Research Working Paper, WEP 10–6/WP73).

Jimenez, E. (1984) *Pricing policy in the social sectors: cost recovery for education and health in developing countries*. Washington, DC, World Bank (CPD Discussion Paper No. 1985–2).

Johnson, O. & Salop, J. (1980) Distributional aspects of stabilization programs in developing countries. *IMF staff papers*, **27**(1): 1–23.

Jolly, R. (1985) *Adjustment with a human face*. New York, United Nations Children's Fund (pamphlet).

Jolly, R. (1988) A UNICEF perspective on the effects of economic crises and what can be done. In: Bell, D. E. & Reich, M. R., ed. *Health, nutrition, and economic crises: approaches to policy in the Third World.* Dover, MA, Auburn House Publishing Co.

Jolly, R. & Cornia, G. A. (1984) *The impact of world recession on children: a study prepared for UNICEF.* Oxford, Pergamon Press.

Katona-Apte, J. (1983) A sociocultural perspective of the significance of sex roles in agriculture. In: *Nutritional impact of agricultural projects.* Rome, International Fund for Agricultural Development.

Kennedy, E. & Cogill, B. (1985) *Effects of the commercialization of agriculture on women's decision making and time allocation.* Paper presented at the annual meeting of the Association of Women in Development, Washington, DC.

Kirkpatrick, C. H. & Diakosavvas, D. M. (1985) Food insecurity and the foreign exchange constraint in developing countries: the case of sub-Saharan Africa. *Journal of modern African studies,* **23**(2): 239–250.

Kumar, S. K. (1979) *Impact of subsidized rice on food consumption and nutrition in Kerala.* Washington, DC, International Food Policy Research Institute (Research Report 5).

Lambert, J. N. (1978) *Does cash cropping cause malnutrition?* Port Moresby, Papua New Guinea, National Planning Office (mimeographed document).

Lau, L. (1975) *A bibliography of macroeconomic models of developing economies.* Palo Alto, Stanford University (mimeographed document).

Lechtig, A. et al. (1975) Effects of food supplementation during pregnancy on birth weight. *Pediatrics,* **56**: 508–520.

Levinson, F. J. (1974) *Morinda: An economic analysis of malnutrition among young children in rural India.* Cambridge, MA (Cornell/MIT International Nutrition Policy Series).

Longhurst, R. (1988) Cash crops, household food security and nutrition. *Institute of Development Studies bulletin,* **19**(2): 28–36.

Mellor, J. W. (1975) *Agricultural price policy and income distribution in low-income nations.* Washington, DC, World Bank (World Bank Staff Working Paper 214).

Montes, M. F. (1987) The impact of macroeconomic adjustments on living standards in the Philippines. *Food and nutrition bulletin,* **9**(1): 39–49.

Pinstrup-Andersen, P. (1983) *Export crop production and malnutrition.* Chapel Hill, University of North Carolina (Occasional Paper Series, Vol. 2, No. 10). Reprinted by International Food Policy Research Institute, Washington, DC.

Pinstrup-Andersen, P. (1985) Food prices and the poor in developing countries. *European review of agricultural economics,* **12** (1/2): 69–81.

Pinstrup-Andersen, P. (1987) Macroeconomic adjustment policies and human nutrition: available evidence and research needs. *Food and nutrition bulletin,* **9**(1): 69–86.

Pinstrup-Andersen, P. (1988) Assuring food security and adequate nutrition for the poor. In: Bell, D. E. & Reich, M. R., ed. *Health, nutrition, and economic crises: approaches to policy in the Third World.* Dover, MA, Auburn House Publishing Co.

Pitt, M. M. & Rosenzweig, M. R. (1983) Health and nutrient consumption across and within farm households. *Review of economics and statistics,* **65**(1): 105–114.

Preston, S. H. (1986) Review of Richard Jolly and Giovanni Andrea Cornia, eds., *The impact of world recession on children. Journal of development economics,* **21**(2): 374–376.

Pyatt, G. & Thorbecke, E. (1976) *Planning for a better future.* Geneva, International Labour Office.

Rabeneck, S. (1982) *The determinants of protein-energy malnutrition among preschool children in Kenya with respect to cash cropping and self-sufficiency in staple food production.* Cornell University, Ph.D. dissertation.

Reutlinger, S. (1987) Poverty and malnutrition consequences of structural adjustment: World Bank policy. *Food and nutrition bulletin,* **9**(1): 50–54.

Rogers, B. L. (1981) *Pakistan: nutrition sector assessment.* Washington, DC, World Bank (mimeographed document).

Rogers, B. L. (1987) Pakistan's ration system: the distribution of costs and benefits. In: Pinstrup-Andersen, P., ed. *Consumer-oriented food subsidies: benefits, costs and policy options.* Baltimore, Johns Hopkins University Press.

Sahn, D. E. (1983) *Malnutrition and food consumption in Sri Lanka: an analysis of changes during the past decade.* Washington, DC, International Food Policy Research Institute.

Sharpley, J. (1988) The foreign exchange content of Kenyan agriculture. *Institute of Development Studies bulletin,* **19**(2): 16–27.

Taylor, L. (1983) *Structuralist macroeconomics.* New York, Basic Books.

Timmer, C. P. et al. (1983) *Food policy analysis.* Baltimore, Johns Hopkins University Press.

Tinker, I. (1979) *New technologies for food chain activities: the imperative of equity for women.* Washington, DC, United States Agency for International Development, Office of Women in Development.

Trairatvorakul, P. (1984) *Effects on income distribution and nutrition of alternative rice price policies in Thailand.* Washington, DC, International Food Policy Research Institute (Research Report 46).

UNICEF (1984) The impact of world recession on children: a UNICEF special study. *State of the world's children 1984.* Oxford, Oxford University Press.

UNICEF (1988a) Redirecting adjustment programmes towards growth and the protection of the poor: the Philippine case. In: Cornia, G. A. et al., ed. *Adjustment with a human face. Vol 2. Country case studies.* Oxford, Clarendon Press.

UNICEF (1988b). Adjustment policies and programmes to protect children and other vulnerable groups in Ghana. In: Cornia, G. A. et al., ed. *Adjustment with a human face. Vol 2. Country case studies.* Oxford, Clarendon Press.

Westcott, G. et al. (1985) *Health policy implications of unemployment.* Copenhagen, WHO Regional office for Europe.

Whitehead, A. (1988) Distributional effects of cash crop innovation: the peripherally commercialised farmers of northeast Ghana. *Institute of Development Studies bulletin,* **19**(2): 59–65.

WHO/World Food Programme (1988) *Structural adjustment, health, nutrition and food aid in the African Region.*

World Bank (1986) *Poverty and hunger: issues and options for food security in developing countries.* Washington, DC.

World Bank (1989) *Research news,* **8**(3).

World Food Council (1985) *Improving access to food by the undernourished.* Report by the Executive Director to the Eleventh Ministerial Session. Paris (document WFC/1985/4).

CHAPTER 3

Agricultural policies

Many agricultural policies have been linked with important health concerns; not all of them can be considered here. This chapter will concentrate on policy and health linkages in four areas: irrigation systems, pesticide use, land policies and resettlement, and agricultural research. Evidence concerning these linkages varies considerably, but in each area enough is available to warrant further study. Many gaps exist, however, in our understanding of how they operate and what policy-makers should do about them. Further work is needed, in particular, on ways of converting a better understanding of them into better health for populations at risk.

Areas not covered here, but which the reader may wish to explore further, include: cropping systems (some crops such as oil palm, coconut, and rubber are associated with scrub typhus and leptospirosis, and there is evidence that multiple cropping may have a positive impact on income and nutrition (Bradley & Narayan, 1987; Francis, 1986; Self, 1987)); the extension of land use into forested ecosystems, which has increased leishmaniasis in Brazil and the southern USSR; livestock development and mechanization (livestock densities have been shown to have an important impact on the epidemiology of some diseases, including Japanese encephalitis associated with pigs in Sri Lanka, while mechanization is associated with malaria in Guyana); the health problems arising from women's participation in agricultural labour; the effects of seasonality of labour on health; and the risks associated with the use of wastewater in irrigation. The health effects of food policies and food pricing policies were considered in Chapter 2, since these measures are used primarily as levers of macroeconomic policy.

Irrigation systems

The most widely recognized links between agriculture and health are those associated with irrigation systems. Because these systems have become an important economic component of agricultural development in many developing countries, evidence of the potential social costs has earned irrigation a high profile along with other vexing "dilemmas of development", including air and water pollution, soil degradation, deforestation, and the depletion of nonrenewable resources. On the positive side, successful irrigation systems will raise income and improve food security, thus increasing the potential for better nutrition and health. With proper planning, the benefits can include better access to safe domestic water supplies and sanitation. On the negative side, however, irrigation systems are often associated with an increased incidence of disease (Tiffen, 1989; Yoder, 1983).

It is universally accepted that irrigation schemes, especially in the tropics, carry a high risk of introducing or increasing the transmission of vector-borne and water-related diseases. The major vector-borne diseases associated with irrigation are schistosomiasis, malaria, onchocerciasis, and Japanese encephalitis. But there are many others; in fact, more than 30 diseases have been linked to irrigation (Hunter et al., 1982; Music, 1987; Tiffen, 1989). Vector-borne disease transmission is aggravated by man-made environmental changes that favour proliferation of the vector, by human behaviour (occupation, choice of dwelling) that increases contact with the vector, and by economic expansion and migration. According to Surtees (1975), six general environmental changes brought about by irrigation systems increase the possibility of vector-breeding: (1) simplification of the habitat; (2) an increase in the area of surface water; (3) a rise in the water table; (4) changes in rates of water flow; (5) a modification of the microclimate; and (6) urban development. The health problems associated with irrigation systems have been extensively reviewed over the past 15 years (McJunkin, 1975; Bradley, 1977; Rosenfield & Bower, 1979; WHO, 1980, 1982; Hunter et al., 1982; Cairncross & Feachem, 1983; Jewsbury, 1984; Mather & That, 1984; Service, 1984; Webbe, 1987).

Hunter et al. (1982) reviewed the negative effects on health of water resource development in Brazil, Côte d'Ivoire, Egypt, Ghana, Indonesia, Kenya, Malaysia, Mali, Nigeria, Paraguay, the Philippines, the Sudan, and Thailand. In all these countries there is some indication that projects to develop water resources have resulted in a higher incidence of vector-borne diseases. Such evidence as they have been able to find, however, relates primarily to malaria and schistosomiasis and, while there have been many studies on irrigation and health, in only a limited number has it been possible to base the conclusions on a comparison of pre- and post-implementation surveys. More frequently, post-implementation surveys are compared with data from areas without water resource development, where malaria or schistosomiasis, for example, is found to be less prevalent. This is, unfortunately, the only kind of evidence that will be available for purposes of comparison until agricultural engineers and other planners provide for pre-implementation health surveys when designing projects.

Although the health risks attached to irrigation schemes are widely recognized, situations where they have successfully influenced the design of such schemes could be better documented. On the whole, baseline data are frequently lacking and post-implementation studies are not often carried out, especially when governments are reluctant to highlight the negative social aspects of costly investments in water resource development (Hunter et al., 1982). Nevertheless, compared with other development initiatives that are likely to have an impact on health, irrigation projects are now more likely to incorporate health objectives or at least to provide for a health assessment, in the planning and implementation process. Another major area of water resource development, namely hydroelectric development, has created similar problems and is discussed in Chapter 5.

Implementation and the spread of disease

The absence of proper drainage systems in irrigation schemes and problems with continuing maintenance are perhaps the two most important factors contributing to the spread of vector-borne disease as a result of irrigation development. Because drainage systems are costly and because the costs of irrigation schemes have been rising steadily over the past 20 years (Levine, 1986; WHO/FAO/UNEP, 1986), drainage construction is often inadequate.

For example, the implementation of a large irrigation scheme on the Cukurova plain of Turkey in the 1970s resulted in a resurgence of endemic malaria in the region. This was due to increased breeding of the vector species in poorly drained ditches which received the run-off of surplus irrigation water. Gratz (1987) found that "there are probably few areas where the cause and effect between agricultural development and increased malaria can be so readily seen as in the Cukurova". He attributed the rise in malaria to "the sequence of construction. . . with very inadequate or. . . no provision for drainage, the increased agricultural activities requiring more and more irrigation and the vast increases in population densities of the main vector in the area, *A. sacharovi*, combined with an influx of migrants, inadequate surveillance activities, and the failure to institute satisfactory control measures in good time." The problems of control were magnified as the working population moved between farms every fortnight so that their employers could avoid liability for welfare contributions.

Another well-known example of irrigation development causing disease is that of the Mahaweli River basin in Sri Lanka, as documented by Wijesundera (1988). The situation might have been different with proper mitigatory measures.

Unfortunately, the cost to the environment and to human health of omitting appropriate drainage systems and other related measures from project plans is usually not taken into account in calculating the internal rate of return (IRR). This calculation is often used by governments and multilateral lending institutions as an indicator of the economic viability of new projects (Tiffen, 1987). With pressure on them to contain costs, planners will be all the more unlikely to provide for improvements in structural design in order to prevent adverse health effects.

Different types of irrigation system (surface, subsurface, oversurface, continuous flow, demand flow, and intermittent flow) and different cycles of water distribution have different effects on the transmission of vector-borne diseases (Goonasekere & Amerasinghe, 1987). There has been evidence from India and Portugal since the early 1940s, for example, that intermittent irrigation in certain circumstances reduces mosquito-breeding and consequently malaria incidence. The irrigation schemes that appear to present the greatest risks of increased transmission of vector-borne diseases are those located where: (1) soils present drainage problems; (2) rice is cultivated; (3) reservoirs are constructed; (4) canals are unlined; and (5) there is compacted settlement or resettlement (Tiffen, 1989).

The differing impact of alternative irrigation systems on health is not the only aspect of the complex relationship between irrigation and health that requires further investigation. The size of irrigation schemes and how and by whom they are run, are also important factors. Hunter et al. (1982) recommended more research on small impoundments since their aggregate impact is probably greater than that of large lakes. This is because they are used by local populations for a variety of purposes, including fishing, water supply, animal watering, irrigation, and flood control; human and animal contact with the water is thus relatively more frequent so that the risks of disease are increased. As international financing is rarely needed for small dams, the likelihood of an environmental health impact assessment at the planning stage is remote. However, "size" is a relative and perhaps misleading term: what is large in Jordan may be small in India. It may be more helpful to speak of "centrally planned" as opposed to "smallholder/community-based" systems.

The latter are the most numerous and the most difficult to monitor in terms of impact on, or risk to, public health (see Tiffen, 1989; FAO, 1987; Small, 1986).

The proper operation and maintenance of irrigation schemes may be critical for health. Small (1986) argued that the participation of farmers in the financing of small irrigation systems would improve their operation and maintenance, and thus benefit health. He recommended devolution of responsibility for running these systems from central government offices to the farmers themselves. It is Small's contention that better cooperation can be achieved between farmers in their communities than between the different government agencies and planners at the central level who have different perspectives and priorities. He also considered that farmers are usually willing to improve their environment if they believe it will lead to better health for themselves and their families (Small, 1986).

Planning and risk assessment

Tiffen (1989) identified four key stages in the planning of irrigation schemes at which cooperation between agencies in different sectors of government is especially important: (1) when terms of reference are drawn up prior to feasibility studies; (2) during the preparation of the feasibility study, when many of the design features important to health will be settled; (3) during the financial negotiations which establish the resources available in different ministries for their necessary role in the scheme; and (4) during the maintenance and monitoring of projects in the operational phase. Studies of how specific projects have proceeded through these phases could provide planners and managers of irrigation development schemes with some valuable insights.

The World Bank has supported a number of case-studies that have attempted to assess the health risks presented by specific projects for the development of water resources in Botswana, India, Kenya, Mali, Morocco, Peru, Sudan, Thailand, and Zambia. Other studies have been carried out by various bilateral assistance organizations and WHO. There are at least two recent "state of the art" collections of case studies of irrigation schemes and their effects on health which deserve mention here: *Health and irrigation*, published in two volumes by the International Institute for Land Reclamation and Improvement (ILRI) (Oomen et al., 1988), and *Vector-borne disease control in humans through rice agroecosystem management*, published by the International Rice Research Institute (IRRI, 1988). The ILRI studies deal with the effects of irrigation projects on health in a wide range of countries, including Brazil, Ghana, Islamic Republic of Iran, Java, Mauritania, Niger, Philippines, Puerto Riço, Sri Lanka, Sudan, and USA, and cover a variety of subjects, including health impact assessment, control measures in reservoirs, and the exploitation of environmental and ecological factors in disease control. The IRRI publication contains articles on a variety of subjects including ecological, entomological, and agronomic management of the environment, planning, engineering, research, impact assessment, and many other matters relating to rice cultivation and the transmission of disease.

The vast amount of work on irrigation systems and their consequences for health has led the joint WHO/FAO/UNEP Panel of Experts on Environmental Management for Vector Control (PEEM) to prepare three documents on vector-borne diseases of relevance to planners in the agricultural and health sectors. Birley (1989) produced a set of guidelines for forecasting the effects of projects for the development of water resources on the prevalence of vector-borne diseases. Tiffen (1989) prepared *Guidelines for the incorporation of health safeguards into irrigation projects through intersectoral co-operation*, which are intended to "alert planners to the linkages between irrigation development and health and to the collaborative intersectoral actions needed to secure the advantages of increased agricultural production and a higher health status in a cost effective way". A third set of guidelines, now in preparation, will deal with the cost-effectiveness of the environmental control of vector-borne diseases.

Pesticide use

Pesticides present a very direct health hazard for rural workers and farmers. The annual number of cases of unintentional acute pesticide poisoning is estimated at over 1 million with an overall fatality rate of 0.4–2% (WHO, 1990), but confidence limits are very wide. To estimate the incidence of, and mortality from, pesticide poisoning and determine the circumstances—environmental contamination, accidental exposure during work, errors in preparation (mixing), failure to use protective clothing, or suicide—is an extremely difficult undertaking. WHO expert committees and panels have gone to great lengths to collect the available data, to consider their accuracy and validity, and to arrive at rough estimates. In addition, there are many studies of the specific effects of particular pesticides on human health. Most of the work on pesticides and health has, however, been limited to confirming the existence of poisoning and investigating the immediate causes (Jeyaratnam et al., 1987; Matos et al., 1987).

In a broad study of pesticide use in the Third World, Bull (1982) compiled information on poisonings (accidental and occupational), pest resistance, environmental damage, pesticide residues in food, and, in particular, the costs and benefits of pesticide use for the Third World poor. Bull suggested that the poor probably bore the brunt of the direct and indirect costs of pesticide use, including environmental damage, crop losses resulting from pest resistance or "secondary" pests, and poisoning.

More research is required on the various occupational hazards associated with long-term exposure to pesticides and acute hazards linked to negligence in their use. WHO and FAO are collaborating on research in this field. WHO is investigating the health hazards, while FAO is examining pesticide registration practices. In 1986, FAO, in collaboration with other international organizations, drew up the International Code of Conduct on the Distribution and Use of Pesticides (FAO, 1986). However, there seems to have been no research to assess the impact of this code on pesticide use.

A recent WHO/UNEP Working Group produced a report on the public health impact of pesticide use in agriculture (WHO, 1990). It covers a wide range of subjects: definition of pesticides, their production and use, evidence of toxic effects, short- and long-term effects of occupational and non-occupational exposure on health, sources and indicators of exposure, populations at risk, implications for public health, approaches to prevention, and research needs. The Working Group offered a series of general recommendations covering control of poisoning, accurate analysis of exposure, and epidemiological research, but did not propose strategies for implementing them.

Lipton & de Kadt (1988) listed four health risks associated with pesticides: direct poisoning, pesticide build-up in the food chain, protein loss due to depletion of fish resources, and development of resistance in nontarget species that may also be important for health (especially in Central America and Mexico). To minimize these risks they recommended better labelling, crop insurance schemes instead of pesticide use, and promotion of more research on pest-resistant crop varieties. Unfortunately, there have been few studies to evaluate the effects on health of specific programmes to implement such alternatives.

Pesticides are only one example of the new health hazards introduced by the modernization of agriculture. Lipton and de Kadt (1988) noted that many other substances widely used on farms (including fertilizers, herbicides, and fungicides) also have implications for health. These have not been sufficiently studied and "the health effects of the great mass of natural and artificial agrochemicals are not well known" (Lipton & de Kadt, 1988; see also Marks, 1984).

Pesticide subsidies

In a study of pesticide subsidies in the Third World, those who benefit from them, and their contribution to the use or misuse of pesticides, Repetto (1985) concluded that such subsidies often resulted in an unnecessary reliance on pesticides when alternative methods of integrated pest management would be safer, cheaper, and more appropriate. Pesticide subsidies are provided in many countries and encourage the overuse of chemicals, depriving governments of funds that could be used to implement and monitor other methods of pest control. Of all the developing countries, only Pakistan (in 1980) has discontinued pesticide subsidies.

In a policy study on pesticide resistance, Dover & Croft (1984) noted that mosquito resistance to major pesticides used in agriculture and public health had developed in 84 countries. This can lead to increased transmission of vector-borne diseases and crop losses affecting income, staple food supplies, and nutrition (see also: Way, 1987; Georghiou, 1987). Repetto (1985) pointed out that "surprising as it may seem, neither the countries maintaining the policies nor the international development agencies have studied what economic and environmental consequences pesticide subsidies have . . . Little is known about the health and environmental consequences of pesticide use . . . little enough is known even about how pesticides are now being used." Moreover, such studies as exist are largely by persons with an *a priori* wish either to defend or to condemn pesticide use, which may bias their research results.

Regulations and enforcement

Studies of regulatory policies for the manufacture, import, marketing, distribution, and use of dangerous pesticides would be particularly useful, as well as studies of their implementation, enforcement, and impact on health. There are few global or regional surveys of pesticide-related legislation, or studies analysing the problems of enforcing pesticide legislation and regulations. Repetto (1985) stated that "although perhaps one-half of the developing countries have basic legislation on the books, in most of them production, use and disposal of pesticides are virtually uncontrolled". Studies of these problems, why they exist, and why they continue are badly needed. While the health dangers of pesticides have been extensively reviewed, it seems that government policies and action to avoid or mitigate these dangers have not. Work in this area would be most valuable and might well begin with a survey of national legislative decisions on pesticide use in key countries.

One notable example of national regulatory action on pesticide use comes from Sri Lanka, where, in 1977, the Government banned the use of malathion and fenitrothion in agriculture, in order to reduce the development of resistance to these insecticides among malaria vectors. Malathion is authorized for use only for indoor spraying as part of malaria control efforts (Herath & Joshi, 1989). However, despite these restrictions, resistance of *Anopheles nigerrimus* and *A. subpictus* to malathion and fenitrothion increased from 1980 to 1987. The selection pressure produced by other pesticides used in rice production in the country may have brought about the increased resistance, and antimalarial spraying may be less important in this respect (Herath & Joshi, 1986, 1989). These studies suggest the need to take into consideration the bionomics of the vector (resting and breeding habits), which determine the nature and extent of selection pressure, in restricting pesticide use for specific purposes.

Training in the safe use of pesticides is sometimes provided in agricultural development projects, but the vast majority of peasant farmers working outside specific projects do not receive any. The present review of the literature has found no case-studies dealing with the impact of such training on farmer/worker behaviour, and thus on the incidence of accidental acute and chronic poisoning. However, there is at least one collection of articles on training issues and pesticide use (Heemstra & Tordoir, 1982); the subjects include education, awareness of health hazards, and licensing procedures for users.

Land policy and resettlement

Policies affecting land tenure may have an indirect but significant impact on the health of rural populations since legal access to, or control over, land is often (though not always) an important determinant of household income. It is assumed here that higher income means better health through greater access to health care, adequate housing, sanitation and hygiene, education, and improved nutrition. Feder & Chalamwong (1986), in a study of land rights in Thailand (see also Feder, 1987), concluded that land titling (the institutionalized registration of land ownership and enforcement mechanisms that protect it) is especially important, since it usually means improved access to credit and working capital and, consequently, higher income-generating capacity. Others have concluded that farmers are more likely to invest in land improvements when ownership is more secure (Feder & Onchan, 1987; Salas et al., 1970; Villamizar, 1984). In addition, Salas et al. (1970) found evidence in Costa Rica of a direct and positive correlation between security of land ownership and income per unit of land. Similar linkages have been demonstrated in Brazil and Ecuador (Inter-American Development Bank, 1986).

A positive connection between size of landholding, income, consumption, and therefore health, has also been reported in a number of countries: Bangladesh (Huffman et al., 1983); El Salvador (Vaughan & Flinn, 1983); Gujarat, India (Wijga et al., 1983; Lipton, 1983); Kenya (FAO, 1984); and Peru (Pines, 1983). For example, one study in Machakos, Kenya, examined the relationship between "landholding per person" and stunting and wasting. The study concluded that there was a strong correlation between "wasting" (or risk of severe malnutrition) and "land poverty" (FAO, 1984).

Other studies have suggested that there are exceptions to the reported relationship between farm size and household income. This relationship is probably weaker when soils are poor, when plots are of inadequate size, and when land is poorly irrigated (Lipton, 1985a; Visaria, 1978). Furthermore, in similar extreme circumstances, landowners may be just as income-poor as non-landowners, owing to the exhaustion or inadequacy of the land, and off-farm income (e.g., wages for labour) may be an equally important part of total income for landowner and non-landowner alike. More important, in many parts of the Third World, "tenancy status" (e.g., as owner, renter, or sharecropper) may have less to do with income than the size of the plot farmed. Therefore, policy-makers cannot assume that "tenancy reform" will result in measurable gains in health status (Lipton & de Kadt, 1988).

Land distribution policies

Land distribution (or redistribution) schemes may increase incomes for the landless rural poor and raise agricultural production, especially of food crops consumed by the poor, in the medium term. On the other hand, where arable land is extremely scarce, land redistribution might reduce employment on large farms and thereby reduce the income of landless labourers (Lipton & de Kadt, 1988). Thus, the impact of land distribution on income, and consequently on health, may well be complex, affecting different population groups in different ways.

The most immediate impact of "land reform" policies on public health may, in some instances, be a negative one, quite apart from any effects it may have on income. Land distribution schemes and policies promoting the colonization of new lands, especially forested areas, may directly increase the risk of major vector-borne diseases, such as malaria and leishmaniasis. A well-documented example is that of the Brazilian Amazon, where the opening of new roads and the distribution of parcels of land to landless farming families have encouraged an enormous influx of farmers, farm labourers, miners, loggers, and others. The major effect on health has been a serious resurgence of malaria, which is concentrated in settlement, mining, and periurban areas across the region (Marques, 1988; Sawyer & Sawyer, 1987; Wilson, 1987).

While much has been written about the economic impact of land tenure policies, few studies have actually documented the links between changes in land tenure and health. It is generally assumed that income changes resulting from changes in land tenancy or land distribution will affect health status—for the better, if income rises, and for the worse, if income declines. Policies affecting access to land, credit, and capital clearly have important economic (and environmental) consequences. But since economic conditions, agrarian structure, and the availability and quality of land vary widely between and within developing countries, it is not feasible to generalize about the degree or direction of the impact of land tenure policies on income and health. It is true, however, that the health consequences of such policies are not routinely considered by policy-makers. This situation might change if policy-makers were routinely confronted with the often costly economic consequences of the health problems associated with agricultural policies (see, for example, Nur, 1986; Wernsdorfer & Wernsdorfer, 1988; and Sawyer & Sawyer, 1987).

Population resettlement

For several decades, evidence has been accumulating on the health problems associated with the resettlement of populations in connection with large-scale agricultural and water resource development schemes, such as those in the Awash Valley of Ethiopia and the Mahaweli region of Sri Lanka, as well as the transmigration schemes in Indonesia. Most of the material relates to increases in vector-borne and communicable diseases with the opening up of new territories, the interaction of previously separated populations, overcrowding, and poor sanitation and infrastructure development (for an extensive discussion of the health risks, see WHO/FAO/UNEP, 1985; see also Sawyer & Sawyer, 1987, on malaria in the Amazon).

Some groups of resettled persons are likely to face greater risks than others. "Scheduled migrants" (those whose movement is determined by planning authorities) are likely to receive more attention than "unscheduled migrants" who choose, or are forced, to move, but without the help of the authorities. Emergency evacuees may experience even more difficulties, given the lack of preparedness to meet their needs. The seasonal resettlement of migrant agricultural workers is often overlooked in planning public health and service programmes (WHO/FAO/UNEP, 1985).

For all groups, resettlement areas may offer less than expected in the way of food production or income generation, thus increasing their vulnerability to health hazards and malnutrition. Even land specifically set aside for gardens and crops may not be of sufficient quality to meet food requirements. Health services may slacken off or lack manpower and resources. Certain institutions, such as the World Bank, apply guidelines on resettlement policy that stress the need to promote the social, economic, and cultural well-being of the populations concerned, as well as providing the basic infrastructure for sanitation and health services. However, there appear to be few empirical studies of the health aspects of specific resettlement ventures or evaluations of the provision of health services in resettlement programmes, even those financed by international agencies. The WHO/FAO/UNEP Panel of Experts on Environmental Management for Vector Control (PEEM) has expressed the view that intersectoral cooperation in resettlement planning is essential for successful health protection and promotion (WHO/FAO/UNEP, 1985). The health and resettlement problems associated with major hydroelectric projects are reviewed in Chapter 5.

Agricultural research, health, and nutrition

In recent years, the International Agricultural Research Centres (IARCs), coordinated by the Consultative Group on International Agricultural Research (CGIAR), have made a substantial effort to incorporate health, nutrition, welfare, and environmental objectives into their agricultural research policies. Attention has been given to analysing the risks associated with agricultural development strategies and assessing the contributions that agriculture can make to improving the health and nutritional status of targeted populations. As these research centres are sponsored by donor nations and international agencies, and work with a number of national research and policy-making institutions, it is likely that their objectives will influence research and programme decisions at all levels.

The International Rice Research Institute (IRRI), based in the Philippines, recently released its work plan for 1990–1994, outlining its goal of improving the "well-being of present and future generations of rice farmers and consumers, particularly those with low incomes" (IRRI, 1989b). The plan is based on the assumption that increasing the productivity of rice-farming systems is essential for "improving nutrition, alleviating hunger, and increasing farm incomes", and that such systems must be environmentally sound and sustainable. In developing a new research strategy, the Institute addressed both the direct and indirect health effects. For example, recommendations are made for research to examine the direct impact of rice production and insecticide use on vector-borne and parasitic diseases, and for studies on the impact of technological change on the income of farmers and consumers (and associated changes in household consumption). The Institute is also concerned with equity in agricultural production and consumption, and intends to increase its support for research programmes that are based on a clear understanding of the needs of target users and beneficiaries.

Issues relating to health status that will be addressed by IRRI in the next decade include: the effects of high-input cropping and climate change on health, income, and the environment; "quantitative understanding of socioeconomic–biophysical–technology interactions and their impact on livelihood, women and the environment"; and the effects of irrigated rice farming on the health of people and farm animals. The development of methods for impact analysis is also on the IRRI agenda. The socioeconomic and environmental costs and benefits of different research strategies will be compared through impact analysis (IRRI, 1989b). It is too early to determine how quickly these research objectives will be implemented, or to predict their long-term effect on health conditions.

Researchers can affect what people grow, sell, and consume through the priority they give to studies on specific commodities and agricultural technologies. Their work may also influence the prices charged for agricultural products, which in turn will affect the income and consumption of both producers and consumers. In the 1980s, high priority was given to research on the staple food crops of developing countries. The health and nutrition of the poor are, therefore, likely to be linked to decisions made by scientists about the kinds of agricultural models and technologies that are developed or adapted, tested in agricultural development projects, and then introduced in the market.

Pinstrup-Andersen (1981) examined some linkages between agricultural and rural development projects and the nutritional status of poor populations. The study looked into the possible effects on nutrition of food output, food prices and income, as well as examining efforts to "incorporate nutritional considerations and goals into the planning and design of agricultural and rural development projects and policies". It found that most national and international agencies were not in a position to deal with those issues, owing to shortcomings in data bases, analytical procedures, supporting research, and institutional frameworks. Pinstrup-Andersen concluded that nutritional considerations should be incorporated into projects at an early stage. In addition, agricultural research should pay much more attention to the nutritional effects of agricultural development.

In an international workshop in 1984, the International Agricultural Research Centres defined four areas of decision-making in agricultural research relevant to nutritional concerns: commodity priorities; desired changes in commodity characteristics; desired technology characteristics; and choice of production systems (Pinstrup-Andersen et al., 1984). The workshop summarized the state of the art in agricultural research and nutritional concerns, as briefly summarized below.

Agricultural researchers need to develop ways of predicting the impact of new crops, crop varieties and farming techniques on the nutritional intake of the poor. However, the necessary information and methods for collecting it are lacking. The workshop held in 1984 by the International Agricultural Research Centres concluded, accordingly, that more study was needed on the diets of malnourished households, on what they produce and consume, and on how consumption responds to changes in prices and incomes caused by technological changes (Pinstrup-Andersen et al., 1984).

In addition, the workshop stressed that "solutions to present nutrition problems should be considered in relation to diet rather than to particular commodities". That is, agricultural research on nutritional problems should take a holistic perspective. For example, when considering changing the characteristics of a particular commodity (e.g., by fortification), this should be weighed against other options, such as changing the composition of the overall diet by encouraging consumption of other commodities that are already available. The workshop's conclusions emphasized the importance of "diagnosing and specifying the nutrition problem separately from a possible solution . . . in order to determine whether changing nutritional characteristics of a commodity or increasing consumption of traditional commodities will be more likely to improve nutrition" (Pinstrup-Andersen et al., 1984).

Conclusion

Four major areas of linkage between agricultural policy and health have been explored in this chapter. This is not intended to be an exhaustive review, and many references have no doubt received inadequate attention. Some of the institutional issues raised in this chapter are being addressed by the joint WHO/FAO/UNEP Panel of Experts on Environmental Management for Vector Control (PEEM) (see Mather & Bos, 1989). The cooperation of major international development agencies, nongovernmental organizations, and national governments will be necessary if the adverse impacts of agricultural development policies are to be effectively reduced.

The work of the Marga Institute in Sri Lanka, in reviewing agricultural policy and health linkages in that country, provides one example of the contribution that local health research can make to the design of appropriate policies and projects. The Institute has produced a general framework for analysis of agriculture–health associations, posed relevant hypotheses for investigation, and produced a preliminary case study on the Mahaweli agricultural development project, revealing changes in nutritional status and vector-borne diseases which may be linked to project activity (Fernando & Gunatilleke, 1989; Perera & Gunatilleke, 1989). This research to inform policy-makers needs to be developed further, and similar efforts need to be pursued in other countries.

Irrigation systems are clearly of importance to public health authorities and to planners seeking to foster agricultural and economic development through development of irrigation. Their effects on health are better understood today than they were two decades ago. Detailed guidelines now exist, based on analyses of the limited data available and on the accumulated and growing experience of specialists in irrigation schemes and in endemic disease control. Engineers tend to be more aware of the problems involved than are agronomists. These guidelines must now be systematically applied, and the resulting changes in health conditions must be measured against the best data that can be acquired from past experience or from areas where such guidelines are not being used. In-depth case studies to monitor the implementation of irrigation schemes and assess efforts to control disease could provide the information needed to bring agricultural policy-makers closer to their counterparts in public health. These studies could attempt to calculate the full costs and benefits of irrigation schemes and assist efforts to ward off unintended effects on public health.

Pesticides, and the use of toxic agrochemicals in general, pose many and diverse threats to public health. People are in danger of direct poisoning from the handling and consumption of these hazardous products. In many areas, pesticide use increases health risks for large numbers of people, because the application of pesticides for agricultural purposes can contribute to the resistance of disease vectors to the chemicals used to control them. The specific effects of pesticides and other agrochemicals on human health are gradually becoming better understood, and health institutions are aware of the need to develop and enforce guidelines to reduce the incidence of unintended poisoning among producers and consumers. Research is needed on how best to implement and enforce existing guidelines. Case-studies reviewing the kinds of legislation on pesticide/agrochemical control that exist in different countries, as well as evaluative studies on the enforcement of this legislation, would fill an important gap in our knowledge of the problem and of what can be done to deal with it.

Studies on the effects of land tenure on income and consumption have been mixed in their conclusions. The literature does not provide any easy generalizations, and the nature and significance of land tenure policy effects on income, consumption, nutrition, and health are very much an open question. Analyses of specific situations and of how land tenure systems function seem to raise more questions than they answer. The legal relationship of farmers to the land may have an important influence on income, consumption, nutrition and/or health status in some areas. It might, however, be of little relevance in others where, for example, soils are severely depleted or where wages for labour off the farm provide a substantial proportion of household income. To understand the relationship between land tenure and health, comparative studies are needed, based on data collected in a variety of economic, ecological, and social contexts. A comparative approach may yield some normative conclusions, and these will probably be limited in scope. At best, such studies might produce classifications of specific types of agrarian systems in which land tenure is, or is not, a significant factor in determining health status. Policy interventions in areas other than land reform or land titling programmes—for example, targeted nutrition programmes, health education programmes, and primary health care programmes—may prove to be politically, socially, and economically more realistic means of improving both productivity and health status.

Policies that play a part in determining priorities for agricultural research can have an impact on land use, production technologies, disease vector propagation, and rural income and consumption. Recently, leading institutions in agricultural research have begun to address directly the effects of agricultural processes on health, nutrition, social welfare and the environment. It may soon be possible—and necessary—to evaluate how these research objectives are being translated into action by research institutes and governments, and how they are influencing agricultural practices at the local level. Several kinds of studies are needed: (*a*) studies of the health and nutritional effects of specific agricultural interventions that have emerged from recent developments in agricultural research; (*b*) studies to determine whether, and how, local research institutions have given increased attention to health concerns in defining their research policies and practices; and (*c*) case studies, in specific countries, of how planners are (or are not) responding to research results that offer new approaches to risk reduction and health promotion in the development of agricultural policies and practices.

References

Birley, M. H. (1989) *Guidelines for forecasting the vector-borne disease implications of water resources development*. Unpublished WHO document WHO/VBC 86.9.

Bottrell, D. G. (1984) Government influence on pesticide use in developing countries. *Insect science and its application*, 5: 151–155.

Bradley, D. J. (1977) The health implications of irrigation schemes and man-made lakes in tropical environments. In: Feachem, R. et al., ed. *Water, wastes and health in hot climates*. London, John Wiley.

Bradley, D. J. & Narayan, R. (1987) Epidemiological patterns associated with agricultural activities in the tropics with special reference to vector-borne diseases. In: *Effects of agricultural development on vector-borne diseases*. Rome, Food and Agriculture Organization of the United Nations (Document AGL/MISC/87.12).

Bull, D. (1982) *A growing problem: pesticides and the Third World poor*. Oxford, Oxfam Press.

Cairncross, S. & Feachem, R. G. (1983) *Environmental health engineering in the tropics: an introductory text*. Chichester, John Wiley.

Dover, M. & Croft, B. (1984) *Getting tough: public policy and the management of pesticide resistance*. Washington, DC, World Resources Institute.

FAO (1987). *Consultation on irrigation in Africa/Policy issues in irrigation development*. Rome, Food and Agriculture Organization of the United Nations (Irrigation and Drainage Paper, No. 42).

FAO (1984) *Integrating nutrition into agricultural and rural development projects; six case studies*. Rome, Food and Agriculture Organization of the United Nations (Nutrition in Agriculture Series, No. 2).

FAO (1986) *International code of conduct on the distribution and use of pesticides.* Rome, Food and Agriculture Organization of the United Nations.

Feder, G. (1987) *Land registration and titling from an economist's perspective: a case study in Thailand.* Washington, DC, World Bank.

Feder, G. & Chalamwong, Y. (1986) *Land ownership security and land values in rural Thailand.* Washington, DC, World Bank (Staff Working Paper No. 790).

Feder, G. & Onchan, T. (1987) Land ownership security and farm investment in Thailand. *American journal of agricultural economics,* **69**(2): 311–320.

Fernando, E. & Gunatilleke, G. (1989) *Agricultural policies and their impact on health.* Colombo, Sri Lanka, Marga Institute.

Francis, C., ed. (1986) *Multiple cropping systems.* New York, Macmillan.

Georghiou, G. P. (1987) The effect of agrochemicals on vector populations. In: *Effects of agricultural development on vector-borne diseases.* Rome, Food and Agriculture Organization of the United Nations (Document AGL/MISC/87.12).

Goonasekere, K. G. A. & Amerasinghe, F. P. (1987) Planning, design and operation of rice irrigation schemes — the impact on mosquito-borne disease hazards. In: *Vector-borne disease control in humans through rice agro-ecosystem management.* Los Baños, Philippines. International Rice Reseach Institute.

Gratz, N. (1987) The effect of water development programmes on malaria and malaria vectors in Turkey. In: *Effects of agricultural development on vector-borne diseases.* Rome, Food and Agriculture Organization of the United Nations (Document AGL/MISC/87.12).

Heemstra, E. A. H. van & Tordoir, W. F., ed. (1982) *Education and safe handling in pesticide application.* Amsterdam, Elsevier.

Herath, P. R. J. & Joshi, G. P. (1986) Factors affecting selection for multiple resistance in *Anopheles nigerrimus* in Sri Lanka. *Transactions of the Royal Society of Tropical Medicine and Hygiene,* **80**: 649–652.

Herath, P. R. J. & Joshi, G. P. (1989) Pesticide selection pressures on *Anopheles subpictus* in Sri Lanka: comparison with two other Sri Lankan anophelines. *Transactions of the Royal Society of Tropical Medicine and Hygiene,* **83**: 565–567.

Huffman, S. et al. (1983) *Pre-school nutrition in Bangladesh.* Baltimore, Johns Hopkins University Press.

Hunter, J. M. et al. (1982) Man-made lakes and man-made disease. *Social science and medicine,* **16**: 1127–1245.

International Fund for Agricultural Development (1983) *Nutritional impact of agricultural projects.* Rome.

Inter-American Development Bank (1986) *Jamaica land titling project feasibility report.* Washington, DC.

IRRI (1988) *Vector-borne disease control in humans through rice agroecosystem management.* Los Baños, Philippines, International Rice Research Institute.

IRRI (1989a) *IRRI: Toward 2000 and beyond.* Manila, Philippines, International Rice Research Institute.

IRRI (1989b) *Work plan for 1990–1994.* Manila, Philippines, International Rice Research Institute.

Jewsbury, J. M. (1984) Small scale irrigation projects and their implications for health. In: *Proceedings of the African Regional Symposium on Smallholder Irrigation.* Wallingford, Overseas Development Unit of Hydraulics Research Ltd.

Jeyaratnam, J. et al. (1987) Survey of acute pesticide poisoning among agricultural workers in four Asian countries. *Bulletin of the World Health Organization,* **65**(4): 521–527.

Levine, R. S. (1986) Assessment of mortality and morbidity due to unintentional pesticide poisonings. Unpublished WHO document WHO/VBC/86.929.

Lipton, M. (1983) *Poverty, undernutrition and hunger.* Washington, DC, World Bank (Staff Working Paper No. 597).

Lipton M. (1985a) *Land assets and rural poverty.* Washington, DC, World Bank (Staff Working Paper No. 744).

Lipton, M. (1985b) *The place of agricultural research in the development of sub-Saharan Africa.* Brighton, Institute of Development Studies (Discussion Paper No. 202).

Lipton, M. & de Kadt, E. (1988) *Agriculture-health linkages.* Geneva, World Health Organization.

McJunkin, R. E. (1975) *Water, engineers, development and disease in the tropics.* Washington, DC, United States Agency for International Development.

Marks, L. (1984) Public health and agricultural practice, *Food policy,* **9**: 131–138.

Marques, A. C. (1988) Main malaria situations in the Brazilian Amazon. SUCAM/Brazilian Ministry of Health (unpublished paper).

Mather, T. H. & That, T. T. (1984) *Environmental management for vector control in rice fields.* Rome, Food and Agriculture Organization of the United Nations (Irrigation and Drainage Paper No. 41).

Mather, T. H. & Bos, R. (1989) *Policies and programmes of governments, bilateral and multilateral agencies and development banks for environmental management in the context of natural resources, agriculture and health development.* Unpublished WHO document, VBC/89.7.

Matos, E. L. et al. (1987) Pesticides in intensive cultivation: effects on working conditions and workers' health. *Bulletin of the Pan American Health Organization,* **21**(4): 405–416 (1987).

Music, S. (1987) *The ex-ante assessment of the health impacts of irrigation projects.* Background paper, Workshop on Assessment of Human Health Risks in Irrigation and Water Resource Development Projects. Paris, World Bank.

Nur, El T. M. (1986) Impact of schistosomiasis and malaria on agricultural productivity in Sudanese irrigated agriculture. Unpublished WHO document TDR/t16/191/SER/1.

Oomen, F. M. V. et al., ed. (1988) *Health and irrigation: incorporation of disease control measures in irrigation; a multi-faceted task in design, construction, operation*. International Institute for Land Reclamation and Improvement, vol. 2, 1988; vol. 1, 1990.

Perera, P. D. A. & Gunatilleke, G. (1989) *Mahaweli project: health policy analysis*. Colombo, Sri Lanka, Marga Institute.

Pines, J. M. (1983) Nutritional consequences of agricultural projects: evidence and response. In: *Nutritional impact of agricultural projects*. Rome, International Fund for Agricultural Development, 1983.

Pinstrup-Andersen, P. (1981) *Nutritional consequences of agricultural projects: conceptual relationships and assessment approaches*. Washington, DC, World Bank (Staff Working Paper No. 456).

Pinstrup-Andersen, P. et al. (1984) *International agricultural research and human nutrition*. Washington, DC, International Food Policy Research Institute.

Repetto, R. (1985) *Paying the price: pesticide subsidies in developing countries*. Washington, DC, World Resources Institute.

Rosenfield, P. & Bower, B. T. (1979) Management strategies for mitigating adverse impacts of water resources development projects. *Progress in water technology*, **11**: 285–301.

Salas, O. et al. (1970) *Land titling in Costa Rica: a legal and economic survey*. San José, University of Costa Rica Law School.

Sawyer, D. & Sawyer, D. (1987) *Malaria on the Amazon frontier: economic and social aspects of transmission and control*. Belo Horizonte, Brazil, Federal University of Minas Gerais/CEDEPLAR.

Self, L. S. (1987) Agricultural practices and their bearing on vector-borne diseases in the WHO Western Pacific Region. In: *Effects of agricultural development on vector-borne diseases*. Rome, Food and Agriculture Organization of the United Nations.

Service, M. W. (1984) Problems of vector-borne diseases and irrigation projects. *Insect science applications*, **5**: 227–231.

Small, L. (1986) *Irrigation financing policies to promote improved operation and maintenance: the role of the farmer*. Unpublished WHO document VBC/87.3.

Stanley, N. F. & Alpers, M., ed. (1975) *Man-made lakes and human health*. London, Academic Press.

Surtees, G. (1975) Mosquitos, arboviruses and vertebrates. In: Stanley, N. F. & Alpers, M., ed. *Man-made lakes and human health*. London, Academic Press.

Taylor, L. (1977) Research directions in income distribution, nutrition, and the economics of food. *Food Research Institute studies*, **16**: 29–45.

Tiffen, M. (1987) *The dominance of the internal rate of return as a planning criterion and the treatment of O & M costs in feasibility studies*. London, Overseas Development Institute.

Tiffen, M. (1989) *Guidelines for the incorporation of health safeguards into irrigation projects through intersectoral cooperation, with special reference to vector-borne diseases*. Unpublished WHO document VBC/89.5.

Vaughan, S. & Flinn, W. (1983) *Socio-economic factors associated with undernourished children: El Salvador rural poor survey, June 1977–July 1978.* Washington, DC, United States Agency for International Development.

Villamizar, F. (1984) *IBD financing in land administration programs.* Paper presented at the International Workshop on Land Tenure Administration, Salvador, Brazil, 1984.

Visaria, P. (1978) *Size of landholding in rural western India.* Washington, DC, World Bank (ESCA-IBRD Working Paper No. 3).

Way, M. J. (1987) Integrated pest control strategies in food production and their bearing on disease vectors in agricultural lands. In: *Effects of agricultural development on vector-borne diseases.* Rome, Food and Agriculture Organization of the United Nations.

Webbe, J. (1987) Planning design and operation of rice irrigation schemes: the impact on schistosomiasis. In: *Vector-borne disease control in humans through rice agro-ecosystem management,* Los Baños, Philippines, International Rice Research Institute.

Wernsdorfer, G. & Wernsdorfer, W. H. (1988) Social and economic aspects of malaria and its control. In: Wernsdorfer, W. H. & McGregor, J., ed. *Malaria: principles and practice of malariology.* Edinburgh, Churchill Livingstone.

Wijesundera, M. de S. (1988) Malaria outbreaks in new foci in Sri Lanka. *Parasitology today,* 4(5): 147–150.

Wijga, A. et al. (1983) Feeding, illness and nutritional status of young children in rural Gujarat. *Human nutrition; clinical nutrition,* 37(14): 255–269.

Wilson, J. F. (1985) *Class and settlement on the Amazon frontier: the case of Ariquemes, Brazil.* Gainesville, University of Florida (Ph.D. dissertation).

Wilson, J. F. (1987) Human issues in malaria control: population, community mobilization, and indigenous peoples (consultant paper for the World Bank).

WHO (1980) *Environmental management for vector control: fourth report of the WHO Expert Committee on Vector Biology and Control.* Geneva, World Health Organization (WHO Technical Report Series, No. 649).

WHO (1982) *Manual on environmental management for mosquito control.* Geneva, World Health Organization (WHO Offset Publication No. 66).

WHO (1986a) *Assessment of mortality and morbidity due to unintentional pesticide poisonings.* Unpublished WHO document WHO/VBC/86.929.

WHO (1986b) *Informal consultation on planning strategy for the prevention of pesticide poisoning.* Unpublished WHO document WHO/VBC/86.926.

WHO/FAO/UNEP (1985) Panel of Experts on Environmental Management for Vector Control (PEEM). *The environmental impact of population resettlement and its effect on vector-borne diseases.* Unpublished WHO document, VBC/85.5.

WHO/FAO/UNEP (1986) Panel of Experts on Environmental Management for Vector Control (PEEM) *Report of the Sixth Meeting*, September 1986. Unpublished WHO document, VBC/86.2.

WHO (1990) *Public health impact of pesticides used in agriculture.* Geneva, World Health Organization.

Yoder, R. (1983) *Non-agricultural uses of irrigation systems: past experiences and implications for planning and design.* London, Overseas Development Institute (Irrigation Network Management Paper 7e).

CHAPTER 4

Industrial policies

Over the last two decades, industrial activity in developing nations has greatly increased. These nations have used a variety of industrial policies to stimulate production and achieve economic gains. As competition rises in world markets, many of them have restructured production in industrial sectors, promoted foreign investment, and encouraged the development of small-scale enterprises.

Industrial growth has also increased the health risks confronting workers and communities in developing countries. Environmental pollution and health hazards have resulted from industrial policies as well as from shortcomings in such areas as financial resources, operational experience, training capacity, information systems, and pollution control technology. These shortcomings have also restricted assessment of the adverse health consequences of industrial development and the establishment of policies for their prevention or control.

This chapter reviews the literature on industrial policies and their consequences for the health of workers and communities in developing countries. Four principal policy areas are reviewed: industrial development policies for specialization, ownership, and siting; occupational health policies; control of industrial pollution; and management of hazardous wastes.

Other important areas (not explored here), in which industrial promotion can conflict with public health objectives, include: preparedness to deal with industrial accidents; health aspects of technology transfer; the contribution of strategies for industrial development in urban areas to traffic congestion, transport accidents, and vehicle pollution; the links between industrial wage rates, income, and nutrition; the health effects of unemployment; the promotion of hazardous consumer products; and the association between industrial development, urbanization, and population growth.

Industrial development policies

Government involvement in industrial development in developing countries is widely viewed as necessary to protect infant industries, and to promote economic growth and exports (Tower, 1986). Intervention often takes the form of protectionist policies which aim at reducing the threat of foreign competition and preserving scarce foreign exchange. Investment incentives, including tax, tariff, and credit benefits, or the provision and pricing of infrastructure, services, and labour, are also among the levers used by governments to promote industrial expansion and diversification, as well as employment and regional economic growth (Leonard, 1988; Galenson, 1984). Few studies of the effects of macroeconomic policies have examined the relationships between industrial policies and health. Given the scope of these policies and the well-attested health hazards posed by industrial operations, a more thorough analysis of these relationships is indicated. There is evidence that some industrial development policies that stimulate economic growth may also increase environmental hazards and counteract measures to improve public health.

In a survey of countries undergoing rapid industrialization, Leonard (1985) examined three areas of industrial policy that can have an important effect on both the generation and control of pollution: industrial specialization, plant ownership, and industrial location. These three areas are considered below in a general review of the literature on the links between industrial development policies and health hazards in developing countries. This overview is followed by a more specific discussion of policies relating to occupational health, pollution control, and waste management. It is important to note that, although epidemiological evidence linking morbidity and mortality to exposure to pollution is not available in most developing countries, the range of possible ill-effects can be inferred from experience in other countries (see, for example, Whittemore, 1981 and Lave & Seskin, 1977, on established links between exposure to air pollution and both respiratory damage and cardiovascular disease).

Industrial specialization

Leonard (1985) argued that policies which encourage specialization in particular industrial sectors can contribute substantially to a rapid increase in pollution hazards. Specialization entails a concentration of capital, human resources, and technology in specific production areas. In order to improve their international competitive position and increase export revenue, developing countries have created incentives for investment in targeted industrial sectors, such as heavy metals, chemical production, and the processing of intermediate products, which present particularly severe health and environmental hazards. Many of these countries have little experience of production or regulation in these areas, having previously concentrated on supplying raw materials or simple manufacturing. Leonard suggested that the increasing global mobility of industry in search of low production costs puts extra pressure on nations undergoing industrial development to create the most favourable conditions for interested multinational firms. The relaxation of environmental laws may be one factor in the negotiations to this end. Thus, specialization may directly contribute to an increase in water and air pollution and in solid wastes, leading to a wide range of health and environmental problems which may offset economic gains.

The net economic and social benefits of industrial specialization may not be properly assessed by government planners or private firms. In an economic analysis of the costs and benefits of the importation of hazardous production facilities, Lee & Lim (1983) suggested that many developing countries inaccurately estimate the domestic economic benefits and fail to measure the costs to efficiency and welfare, notably those resulting from increased pollution. They considered that, before promoting foreign pollution-intensive industrial investment, policy-makers should examine four key concerns: wage gaps, transaction costs, possible environmental damage, and the nature of market distortions. To this list one might add the cost to environmental health and the associated losses in productivity.

Even when government and industry are aware of the potential environmental and health risks, they may lack the interest, resources, or capacity to provide for adequate protection against them. Lepkowski (1987) asserted that developing nations were encouraging the "chemicalization" of industrial production without giving appropriate priority to the promotion and regulation of health and safety. In a number of developing countries undergoing rapid industrialization, the stringency and scope of environmental health and safety regulations are increasing, but their enforcement remains weak. Moreover, because one population group may reap the benefits while another suffers the health consequences, the former group having a key role in decision-making, the assessment of risks may not be wholly objective.

Many health and environmental analysts predicted the proliferation in the 1970s and 1980s of "pollution havens" in developing countries, as a result of the application of strict environmental health and safety regulations in the industrialized countries (Castleman, 1985; Jasanoff, 1985; Lee & Lim, 1983). There is little evidence that this has taken place on the scale predicted, although some developing countries have promoted investment by loosening environmental controls (Leonard, 1988; Pearson, 1987; Castleman, 1987). Overall, the decision to invest tends to be based on factors other than the nature of the environmental regulations in force (Leonard, 1988; Pearson, 1987; Levenstein & Eller, 1985; Galenson, 1984). "For most multinational industries, location decisions are usually based on factors such as labour costs, tax incentives, market conditions, political stability, and the availability of transportation and adequate infrastructure" (Leonard, 1985).

For some pollution-intensive industries, however, environmental factors may play an important role in the decision to operate in a developing country. Industries that prove unprofitable in industrialized countries may find relocation to developing nations attractive, because they are able to avoid costly health and safety measures in their new locales (Leonard, 1985; Castleman, 1987). It has been suggested that the loosening of safety standards by Union Carbide in its plant in Bhopal, India, resulted from efforts to cut back expenses and increase production in the financially troubled factory (Gladwin, 1987).

Another feature of industrial specialization that may intensify risks to health and the environment is the creation of geographical areas where extraordinary opportunities exist for investment. Numerous countries in South-East Asia, Latin America, and the Caribbean have developed export processing zones to attract foreign-owned firms specializing in such areas as chemical and raw-material processing, clothing manufacture, and electronics assembly, the final products being exported to foreign markets. Unlike some industrial estates, these areas are not designed for purposes of pollution control or concentration, but to provide more attractive sites for foreign industry. Preferential tariff, rent, tax, and infrastructure arrangements, reduced regulation, and low-cost labour are offered to multinationals (see Warr, 1989). The factories often create new health risks for workers, particularly women, as will be discussed in the section on occupational health policies (page 71). Because these zones concentrate industrial activity and attract a large labour pool, they also present potentially serious risks for residential communities and the environment through air and water pollution, if they are uncontrolled.

Plant ownership

The diversity of industrial ownership patterns in developing nations creates a variety of regulatory problems for governments (Leonard, 1985). Public enterprises, joint ventures, and industries owned by multinational firms operate differently, and health and environmental hazards result in part from variations in economic, technological, and management choices. Inadequacies in government regulation and enforcement may increase the incidence of industrial diseases and accidents. However, there has been insufficient research to ascertain whether ownership status has significantly influenced the application of health and safety measures in industrial firms or the effectiveness of government health and safety regulations.

Although they tend to be smaller and less pollution-intensive, domestically owned undertakings may be more difficult to regulate than industries owned by multinational firms (Leonard, 1985; Pearson, 1987). The production processes they adopt—e.g., in mineral processing—may be less sophisticated and may not incorporate pollution reduction techniques. Michaels et al. (1985) suggested that the rapid growth of domestic industries in Latin America posed more substantial occupational health risks than the importation of hazardous industries. In India, numerous hazardous chemicals and materials, such as benzidine, asbestos, DDT, and polychlorinated biphenyls, are used in local industries, although they have been restricted or banned in industrialized nations (Lepkowski, 1987). In many developing nations, domestic firms have become the principal producers of products banned elsewhere in the world.

Older, and thereby often more hazardous, industrial operations in developing countries are frequently owned and operated by domestic firms. Multinational firms tend to shut down old facilities rather than incur the cost of upgrading technology and installing pollution control devices. Domestic firms rarely have the operational or financial flexibility to consider shutting down and frequently lack the capital for imported pollution control devices (Leonard, 1985). Older and smaller firms may also lack the capital required for necessary repairs or the replacement of hazardous parts, in turn increasing the likelihood of accidents (Asogwa, 1987).

The political context can affect the impact of government regulations on domestic as compared with foreign firms. Government officials with connections in local industry may often have the power to relax controls on local firms but do not have the same allegiance to foreign-controlled industries (Leonard, 1985). Since most pollution control standards are set on a case-by-case basis, they may be more stringent with regard to multinational firms. For multinational firms with newer operations, the benefits of production in low-cost developing countries may outweigh the costs of the technology adaptation, pollution control, and safety measures required to meet government standards. Therefore, the compliance of multinational corporations with government regulations may be more certain than that of local firms (Pearson, 1987; Leonard, 1985). However, enforcement of regulations often remains in the hands of local officials who may lack the resources to perform the task adequately and may be prone to corruption. The possible effects of local corruption on environmental regulation remain relatively unexplored.

In some areas, there is strong evidence of "double standards" on the part of multinational firms with regard to plant design, production processes, and the application of health and safety measures in operations in the home country as compared with operations in developing countries. The existence of such double standards is well documented in the case of the Union Carbide accident in Bhopal, India (see Castleman & Navarro, 1987). There is evidence that the corporation failed to anticipate hazards, equip the plant properly, inform workers, control hazardous conditions, and comply with its own safety standards (Gladwin, 1987). In Brazil, multinational firms continued to produce asbestos materials in the 1980s without providing safety training for workers, protective equipment, or public information, in spite of the stringent precautionary measures regarding asbestos adopted in industrialized nations (Berman, 1986). In most developing nations, asbestos remains one of the cheapest and most readily available building materials; and hazardous pesticides have become ubiquitous in agricultural production. The incentives for governments to maintain the domestic supply of these products may outweigh the incentives to restrict their production.

A variety of government regulations, unrelated to environmental health, may inadvertently encourage foreign industry to reduce safety measures. In an analysis of the Bhopal disaster, Gladwin (1987) contended that the government's import restrictions, local ownership requirements, promotion of labour-intensive technology, and laxity of inspection all contributed to the development of the hazardous conditions that led to the release of the chemical. The production process in the Union Carbide plant required supervision by highly trained specialists and automated safety instruments, but became the responsibility of a poorly trained and inexperienced workforce which was unable to predict or prevent the accident.

Some studies suggest that public regulatory systems may be more important than industry ownership in influencing action or inaction on pollution control. Pimenta (1987) concluded that in Brazil "neither legislation nor government behavior separates [multinationals] from domestic firms, and the main issue is more effective pollution control, regardless of business ownership". Pimenta suggested that the organization of government responsibilities, especially as regards giving sufficient powers to local officials, was a critical factor in monitoring and regulating private firms, whether domestic or foreign-owned. The legal and illegal use of powers will also influence the effectiveness of pollution control measures. There are few country analyses dealing with these and related aspects of institutional structure and policy in respect of pollution control.

Some governments have succeeded in reducing industrial risks through cooperation with multinational firms. In Brazil, the industrial district of Cubatao, which has high pollution levels and a heavily concentrated population, has recently adopted an accident/emergency preparedness system involving both the public and private sectors. Multinational and local industrial firms are seeking to ensure that there are clear procedures and adequate training within chemical plants (Leonard, 1986; Pimenta, 1987). In São Paulo, the pollution control agency has provided loans to enable industries to meet federal and state quality standards for air and water (Thomas, 1985). Careful examination of the interaction of multinationals, policy-makers and regulatory officials in such initiatives might provide useful lessons for policy development in the future.

Location of industries

In stimulating economic growth, some countries have encouraged a dispersion of industry, whereas others have encouraged concentrated industrial development. Interest in controlling pollution has been a contributory factor, but rarely the decisive one, in the choice of approach (Leonard, 1985). When providing incentives for industrial siting, government policy-makers have often ended up making trade-offs between economic and environmental interests, one consequence being increased pollution.

To counteract this trend, governments are taking steps to implement firmer environmental regulations for industrial siting and emissions. For example, in 1980 the Federal Government in Brazil gave power to state and local authorities to regulate zoning on the basis of pollution criteria. São Paulo, where pollution problems are especially severe, has put strict zoning and licensing requirements into effect in order to meet quality standards for air and water. While hazardous levels of pollutants continue to be emitted by established industries, the above measures have helped to limit new sources of pollution, and some recently established industries have chosen to develop operations in less pollution-ridden locations outside the metropolitan area (Thomas, 1985). Unfortunately, few other countries have as yet established effective guidelines for industrial siting. Even fewer appear to have incorporated health objectives into plans for regional development.

Industrial dispersion policies are most often viewed as means of distributing resources across regions, increasing markets, expanding employment opportunities, and diverting population growth from overcrowded urban centres (Hamer, 1985). In most developing countries, the concentration of commercial activity, supply markets, communications technology, transport, and other basic items of infrastructure in a few major cities attracts industrial firms and may defeat government measures to encourage dispersion (Hamer, 1985; Leonard, 1985; Galenson, 1984). The concentration of wealth and political power in urban areas also militates against the siting of industries in rural areas, despite the economic benefits of choosing areas where there is an abundance of low-cost labour (Tower, 1986). Mispricing of transport, services, and infrastructure can also favour siting in core regions for reasons of efficiency (Vining, 1985; Tower, 1986). The distribution of industry naturally affects the growth rates of urban populations, so that industrial and housing policies (see Chapter 6) are linked.

Additional government incentives for dispersion, such as the guaranteed provision of infrastructure and services, are generally required to entice industry away from the main cities (Hamer, 1985). In São Paulo, for example, more than zoning requirements or pollution taxes and fines were used to encourage the dispersion of polluting industries. Major state investments were made to improve local infrastructure and services so that they met industrial needs (Townroe, 1983). However, the ability of many developing countries to offer such incentives may be limited by lack of resources.

Some countries (such as Brazil, Colombia, Mexico, Republic of Korea, and Thailand) have created "industrial estates", which are located away from major urban areas in places where industrial growth is more manageable and "economies of scale in the construction of infrastructure and in the provision of waste disposal" are possible (Leonard, 1985). However, the economic benefits have been partially offset by new health hazards created by the estate or industrial district itself. In Japan, the promotion of large-scale industrial complexes in the 1950s and 1960s has been linked to high levels of pollution and related health problems (Huddle & Reich, 1975).

Similar problems are now being recorded in many developing countries. In the industrial district of Cubatao, Brazil, where 23 major industrial plants and numerous small operations are concentrated, serious health problems, including an elevated neonatal mortality rate, birth deformities, and a high prevalence of respiratory disorders, have been associated with high levels of water and air pollution (see Findley, 1988; Pimenta, 1987; Thomas, 1981). Frequent industrial explosions and fires in the area have led to the temporary, and in some cases permanent, displacement of nearby residents, causing additional welfare effects. Near the Rio Guanabara Bay in São Paulo, where many industries have been located so that they can discharge their effluents into the ocean, the regional environmental agency has found an association between the area's infant mortality rate of 200 per 1000 live births and pollution levels in the bay (Ledec & Goodland, 1984). In Malaysia, large-scale industrial projects have been criticized for displacing thousands of households and destroying communities, probably with severe repercussions on health and social welfare, and the industrial area of Perai has produced heavy particulate pollution related to the processing of minerals and fossil fuels (Rajeandran & Reich, 1981). Systematic analysis is needed of the association between the development of industrial districts, pollution levels, and health problems.

The rapid expansion of urban areas has further complicated efforts to deal with environmental and health problems arising from the location of industries. Industries that were constructed five or ten years ago beyond city limits have now become part of, and have contributed to, urban sprawl. Given scarce resources and limited transport facilities, new migrants and the low-wage labour force attracted to urban areas may have no alternative but to settle in dangerous proximity to the plants. In the long run, the establishment of industrial growth zones away from urban centres may inadvertently create major health hazards. The 6000–20 000 deaths and over 15 000 injuries caused by the methyl isocyanate emission in Bhopal were due in part to the concentration of settlements around and close to the plant. Despite increased government regulation of industrial production and the use of hazardous substances in India since the disaster, there has been little improvement in policies for the siting of industries or land use (Rosencranz, 1988). Squatter settlements are likely to continue to proliferate around industrial plants, posing significant hazards for the residents. The avoidance of public health emergencies in the future will depend not only on active efforts by government and industry to improve the control of industrial pollution, but also on better industrial location policies and public housing initiatives.

Thus, the choice of sites for both concentrated and dispersed industries can create health hazards relating to production processes and the disposal of wastes. A comparative study of the costs and benefits of siting alternatives, including anticipated clean-up costs, would be useful for policy-makers. In 1980 the United Nations Environment Programme published *Guidelines for assessing industrial environmental criteria for siting of industry*. It may be an appropriate time to evaluate the effects of such international or national guidelines on the design and implementation of industrial development policies. The establishment in 1980 of industrial zoning laws by national, state, and local authorities in Brazil may serve as an important example for other nations (see Findley, 1988).

Additional empirical evidence is required to assess the associations between health conditions and government policies for industrial development with respect to specialization, ownership, and siting patterns. Studies of the health effects of pollution in developing nations still have a long way to go, and predictions of the nature and seriousness of the effects of industrial development strategies on health are still rudimentary. Country-specific analyses of the linkages involved and evaluations of policy implementation would assist decision-makers in identifying the policy adjustments that will effectively reduce health hazards.

Population size, geographical factors, and industrial characteristics all have a role in determining the severity of the health hazards posed by the location of industries. Thomas (1981) developed a method based on cost-benefit analysis to assess area-specific pollution control measures in São Paulo, Brazil. Working with researchers from the University of São Paulo, and in collaboration with the State of São Paulo environmental agency, CETESB, Thomas assessed the welfare benefits, in terms of reduced mortality, and the effects on production costs of local regulations for the control of industrial pollution. Thomas's study also predicted the effects of pollution control measures on decisions concerning the siting of industries. It appeared that regulation would affect production costs and, in turn, industrial output. The study concluded that spatially variable policies of pollution abatement were preferable to outright industrial zoning or licensing, and that such policies could divert production away from highly polluted areas. Region-specific cost-benefit research of this kind can assist policy-makers in introducing pollution control measures that will prompt socially beneficial decisions on the location of industries.

Occupational health policies

The industrial development strategies discussed above are likely to have an influence on occupational health and pollution control policies, or the lack thereof, and consequently on health. Unfortunately, even where explicit policies exist to protect workers and residents in industrial areas, their implementation remains an unattained objective in most cases. The following sections explore the literature on major occupational and pollution-related health problems in developing countries, and discuss policy measures that have been taken to deal with them. However, there has been only limited research on the political or social contexts in which such problems develop. Most of the associations suggested here between industrial development policies, health consequences and health protection accordingly need to be investigated further.

With the expansion of industrial operations in developing nations, there is an overlap between those continuing to suffer from parasitic diseases, respiratory infections, and malnutrition and those that have experienced development of illnesses and disability associated with new work settings and processes. Rapid industrialization may in fact intensify existing health problems in developing countries (El Batawi, 1981). Disease and illness among workers in many developing countries have been due to exposure to common industrial materials such as vinyl chloride, lead, asbestos, chromium, and silicon dust, and to noise pollution. Occupational cancers and respiratory problems have been associated with elevated rates of tuberculosis and other diseases common in low-income communities. Health problems frequently associated with industrial operations in developing and industrialized nations include obstructive respiratory diseases and irritation due to inhalation of gases and vapour, heavy metal poisoning, low-back pain, byssinosis, chronic bronchitis and silicosis, occupational dermatitis and cancers, noise-induced hearing loss, and a range of accident-induced disabilities (Durvasula, 1988; Phoon, 1983; El Batawi, 1981).

Although texts on occupational health refer briefly to the occupational health problems of developing countries, few in-depth studies of the subject exist (Christiani et al., 1990; Rossiter & El Batawi, 1987; Phoon & Ong, 1985; Phoon, 1983; El Batawi, 1981). Reviews of national or regional health problems touch only briefly on occupational health. While there is a growing body of epidemiological studies in this area, they cover only a limited range of industries and occupational diseases, and problems relating to the availability, validity, and completeness of data abound.

Some of the most prevalent and severe occupational diseases and risk factors in developing countries have yet to be adequately investigated. "Topics studied thus far have been principally concerned with the 'old' occupational diseases. There have been few attempts to study the effects of newer technology which is well represented in developing countries . . . There is relatively little on chemical toxicity other than heavy metals and pesticides or on occupational cancer or neurotoxicity" (Christiani et al., 1990). Especially needed is research on the mental health problems associated with work stress, automation, rigid production systems, and shift work, among other features of the industrial working environment in developing countries (de Rosen, 1987). The methodological and logistic problems associated with research on mental health in the workplace have meant that this field of study has only recently started to expand, even in industrialized countries. Thus, the empirical findings available to policy-makers may not reflect the full scope and severity of the occupational health problems with which workers are confronted.

In many developing countries, inadequate information creates major obstacles to the effective assessment of occupational health problems and the formulation of policies to deal with them. Researchers and regulatory officials often lack access to records held by private industry, multinational firms being particularly difficult to monitor. Even when data are available, under-reporting remains a major problem (Phoon, 1983). Data can also be difficult to compile and analyse because of the multiplicity of government departments involved in dealing with workers and industrial development (Christiani et al., 1990). The responsibility for occupational health programmes is often divided between departments or ministries, and there is little communication between public health authorities, occupational health specialists, and industry analysts, the result being significant problems of overlapping and gaps in coverage (Phoon, 1983). Administrative problems of this kind can significantly limit the scope and effectiveness of industrial regulation.

In most country studies of occupational health, government standard-setting and legislative issues are dealt with only briefly, and recommendations for improved policies and enforcement are rarely well developed. It is often considered that malnutrition, communicable diseases, and population growth are more urgent issues than occupational health and require greater attention (Phoon, 1983). Studies of occupational health problems, however, can provide important insights into the direct and indirect associations between industrial policies and health. The identification of hazard-creating policies which are amenable to change should be a priority.

Small-scale industry, agriculture, and the informal sector

While occupational health research in developing countries concentrates to a large extent on conditions in large factories or mines, only an estimated 15–20% of the labour force in those countries is employed in large urban enterprises (Phoon, 1983). Approximately 60–85% of the workers are employed in agriculture, small industries, or other small enterprises (Forssman, 1981), and the number is growing. Flax processing, textiles, garment and footwear manufacture, rubber-curing, gem-polishing, foundry work, and scrap-processing are among the hundreds of expanding small industries in urban and rural areas. Workers in small-scale industries, agriculture, and fisheries, migrant labourers, and those employed in the informal sector face occupational risks that are distinct from those of urban industrial workers and perhaps of even greater intensity (Christiani et al., 1990; Phoon, 1983).

As noted in Chapter 3, the mechanization and "chemicalization" of agriculture and the growth of agricultural processing operations in developing countries have exacerbated the acute and chronic health problems confronting workers in this sector. These problems include pesticide poisoning, byssinosis, asthma, injury, and long-term disability (Christiani et al., 1990; Rossiter & El Batawi, 1987; Noweir, 1986; Blanc, 1984). Most large-scale agricultural operations, such as plantations, provide formal health services for workers and are subject to frequent health and safety inspections, especially if operated by multinational firms. However, labourers in small agricultural operations rarely have access to health services, and their employers may not be subject to inspection or enforcement of regulations. Similarly, small-scale industries and activities in the informal sector often lack the resources, interest, or political pressure to respond to the health needs of workers. Nogueira (1987), in a study of accident prevention in Brazil, noted that while combined public and private efforts in the industrialized south of the country have led to significant reductions in accident rates, the incidence of serious injuries continues to be high in agricultural undertakings and small industries in the north and north-east. Federally sponsored, but region-specific, initiatives for the promotion of occupational health and safety are considered necessary to iron out the differences.

China provides an example of a policy-based increase in small industries which preceded adequate provision for occupational health. In the late 1970s and early 1980s, China's industrial policy promoted the development of light industries, which were viewed as critical to economic growth because of the limited financial and technical input required. The Government gave special attention to the expansion of industries based on the model of the collective farm. In China, 17.5% of the national industrial output in 1980 came from small-scale cooperative operations involving nearly seven million workers (Christiani, 1984). Despite the rapid growth in the industrial workforce, there was no related expansion in the provision of health personnel to help meet the needs of industrial workers. In most areas of the country, there are few trained occupational health personnel, which precludes both an adequate assessment of health problems and the provision of occupational health services and safety measures for light industries. Even where there are trained specialists, bureaucratic inertia and neglect may inhibit action in these areas. Workers in collective operations lack the benefits, including worker compensation, afforded to those in state enterprises and have limited access to health services. New health and safety regulations are being developed in China for smaller industries, but there are numerous obstacles to their effective enforcement. These include the difficulty of regulating state-owned enterprises when it is not always clear in whose hands the ultimate authority rests (Quinn et al., 1987).

Similar problems face those employed in small-scale enterprises elsewhere in the world. El Batawi & Husbumrer (1987) conducted surveys on health conditions in small and medium-sized factories on an industrial estate in Thailand and concluded that the prevalence of disease was higher in the smaller plants. As a result of this study, the Government is striving to pay greater attention to occupational health problems in primary health care training, increase regulatory activities, and reduce occupational hazards. Similarly, studies of occupational health conditions and policies in Brazil (Nogueira, 1987) and in Nigeria (Asogwa, 1987) demonstrated that injury rates were higher for workers in small-scale industrial undertakings than for those in large firms. Conditions may be even more extreme than current injury statistics suggest, as data collection and reporting requirements are generally poorly enforced in small firms. In Nigeria, the enforcement of health and safety measures in small firms is limited, owing to the official definition of a factory. Firms are visited by inspectors only if they employ at least 10 persons, but the vast majority employ no more than 6 or 7 and therefore go uninspected (Asogwa, 1987).

For those employed in the informal sector, job security is likely to be more important than industrial hygiene or the provision of worker benefits and insurance (de Rosen, 1987; Michaels et al., 1985). Therefore, the demand by the labour force for occupational safety and health measures is not strong in this sector. The enforcement of existing standards can be particularly difficult within the informal sector, owing to the temporary nature of many businesses and their unregistered status (WHO, 1988). The absence of technical expertise or funds for the purchase of safety equipment can also limit compliance with regulations in small enterprises (see Noweir, 1986).

In rural areas, profound social and environmental changes accompany land and water resource development, as well as investment in small industries. These changes have been linked to the increased transmission of a whole range of diseases, including malaria, cholera, filariasis, trypanosomiasis, and leishmaniasis (WHO/FAO/UNEP, 1985; USAID, 1980; Christiani et al., 1990). Because most rural development projects attract or actively recruit migrant labourers who interact with local populations, increases in the incidence of sexually transmitted diseases, and in the transmission of infectious diseases, are common. The poor quality of the housing provided for workers also increases their vulnerability to disease. Private or public industrial development projects may have similar effects on the disease profile of the surrounding communities (USAID, 1980). Government policies that encourage such projects, without requiring appropriate planning and provision of services, may contribute inadvertently to an increase in the health risks just outlined.

High-risk groups: children and women

Children are believed to make up a growing percentage of the workforce in the informal sector in many developing countries (Christiani et al., 1990). In most countries, child labour results from failure to implement protective policies, particularly in small industries, rather than from policies that encourage such labour. There are differing views on the definition of child labour and its worldwide extent, with estimates of the number of children involved ranging from 50 to 300 million (Pitt, 1985).

Research shows that child workers are more susceptible than adult workers to communicable diseases, occupational illnesses, and impaired function, and their health problems may be compounded by malnourishment and poverty-related disease (WHO, 1988; Christiani et al., 1990; Pitt, 1985). Toxic exposure levels and the incidence of occupational accidents in this group have been found to be high, because of the children's lack of training and work-site experience (Pitt, 1985; Michaels et al., 1985; Burra, 1988). Child labour may also have long-term indirect effects on child growth and development (Pitt, 1985). WHO recently produced a *Training manual on research and action methodologies and techniques concerning the health of working children* (WHO, 1988) which reviews the health problems of child workers and provides guidance on data-handling, epidemiological and qualitative methodology, survey design and analysis, and health assessment techniques. The manual also offers a framework for research, examines the role of primary health care, discusses international and national policies on child labour and the problems involved in their implementation, and offers methods for the evaluation of measures taken.

While efforts to reduce child labour are increasing throughout the world (WHO, 1988; Shah, 1985), the influx of children into the workforce does not appear to be lessening, as economic crises increase the need for additional household income. The enforcement of child labour regulations remains a major challenge for many reasons such as poor understanding of the law on the part of government officials and employers, difficulties in confirming children's ages, a shortage of labour inspectors, and the proliferation of unregistered enterprises (WHO, 1988; Pitt, 1985). WHO recommends that countries adopt a multi-pronged approach to the problem, involving: regulatory action, public information, enhanced provision of primary health care services, nutrition supplementation, and efforts to improve working conditions.

In a recent analysis of industrial development in sub-Saharan Africa, Packard (1989) noted that the literature on occupational health paid scant attention to the special health risks facing women workers in the informal sector. Serious and unreported health hazards have been found in factories and small subcontracting shops primarily employing women, and also among women doing piecework at home (Beneria & Roldan, 1987). As well as supplementing family income, women in most countries are solely responsible for the tasks of family care and household maintenance. It has been suggested that this "double burden" increases women's susceptibility to disease, accidents, and stress in the workplace (Singh & Kelles-Viitanen, 1987).

In spite of the limited research on the occupational health problems suffered by women workers in developing countries, a number of studies have revealed important relationships between women's work and illness. For example, research on women workers in a district of the United Republic of Tanzania found that those performing heavy agricultural tasks were at a higher risk of having babies with low birth weights than women engaged in less strenuous work (Kamuzora, 1986). While there has been no confirmation of a causal association between strenuous work during pregnancy and low birth weight in offspring, the existence of such an association is considered "potentially important and modifiable" (Kramer, 1987; Ashworth & Feachem, 1985).

Research on breast-feeding, a major factor in reducing infant diarrhoea, suggests that working women are less likely to breast-feed (Van Esterik & Greiner, 1981; Feachem, 1986). Easier access to crèches, maternity leave, and special breaks for women workers can make breast-feeding a feasible option, but the costs of such benefits, unless covered by employers, may preclude their widespread adoption (Phillips et al., 1987). Experience in countries such as Brazil suggests that regulations making benefits of this kind mandatory may inadvertently lead to a reduction in the employment of women by encouraging discriminatory hiring practices. A systematic comparative evaluation of such benefits could influence the future design and application of measures that will help to improve breast-feeding practices without creating employment problems or financial difficulties for women workers. Epidemiological analysis is also needed to assess what changes in working practices may lead to the greatest improvements in maternal and child health.

Plants in export processing zones tend to employ young unmarried women, who form the cheapest pool of unskilled labour and are considered particularly suitable for precise, repetitive tasks in such areas as the mass production of garments and electronic equipment. These workers commonly work in the zones for only a couple of years, leaving to be married or to move back to their home communities. Industries are believed to rely on this rapid turnover of labour to avoid wage increases and demands for improved working and living conditions in the zones (Sun, 1989). While the wages are low by international standards, they are usually far more than the alternatives open to the young workers would provide, so that they are discouraged from complaining and risking dismissal. Because the industries involved are highly mobile, governments are not keen to impose new regulations, fearing a flight of industry. As a result, improvements to plants are infrequent, and the enforcement of safety regulations may be lax (Sun, 1989; Hovell et al., 1988).

The health problems reportedly associated with employment on the production lines in export processing zones have included acute chemical poisoning, chronic conjunctivitis, eye-strain, migraine headaches, rheumatism, arthritis, brown lung disease, and fatigue resulting from the intensity of the work and the working hours—in most zones, 45–50 hours per week is common; in some, overtime, often unregulated, brings the working week up to 65–70 hours (Sun, 1989; Singh & Kelles-Viitanen, 1987; Pineda Ofreneo, 1987; ILO, 1985; Fuentes & Ehrenreich, 1984). However, the causal relationships between illness in workers and factory conditions and practices have not been adequately demonstrated. Few formal epidemiological studies have been carried out, as access to plants is limited, health and injury information is often poorly documented, the identification of control or comparison groups is difficult, and other methodological problems are liable to arise.

Some research, however, suggests that the overall health level of factory workers in export processing zones may in fact be considerably higher than that of their counterparts employed outside the formal sector. The higher incomes factory workers receive can mean improved consumption for themselves and their families, to whom most migrant workers send money (ILO, 1985). A recent household-based study in the export processing zone in Tijuana, Mexico, investigated whether women factory workers had higher morbidity rates than other women in the same low-income community (Hovell et al., 1988). The researchers found that these workers suffered from no more short-term illness (as measured by self-reported symptoms) than other women working outside the home and from less illness than women working exclusively in the home. The findings suggested that, thanks to their higher income combined with health and social security benefits to which their counterparts lacked access, the women factory workers had a lower risk of poverty-related illness. However, it was noted that many major occupational diseases and illnesses have long latency periods, that the plants are still relatively new, and that most of the workers are young with little or no previous manufacturing experience. Thus it may be too early to assess the health effects of employment in these government-supported industrial areas.

Few industrial regulations dealing with problems of reproductive health, such as spontaneous abortion, depressed libido, and congenital malformations, have as yet been applied in either industrialized or developing countries. A study produced by the Office for Technology Assessment of the United States Congress (1985) has explored the various occupational hazards for men and women in this area, as well as the appropriate risk assessment techniques and the existing legislation on the subject, in order to provide information on which future policy can be based. The principal hazards suspected of impairing reproductive functions include: workplace chemicals; metals; ionizing and non-ionizing radiation; physical factors such as temperature, noise, and vibration; infectious diseases; life-style factors; ingestion or absorption of drugs; and overexertion and stress. The report emphasized that there is "no reliable estimate as yet of the basic measures of reproductive risk in the workplace".

Of critical importance for the development of adequate legislation to protect the reproductive health of workers is improved risk assessment leading to appropriate risk management. The USA has succeeded in restricting the use of some chemicals shown to be linked to severe reproductive malfunction—a ban on dibromochloropropene, used in pesticides, is one example. The international exchange of study results and regulatory information will be essential if risks are to be substantially reduced. However, to make accurate choices as regards risk management, the assessment process must examine intervening genetic, environmental, and behavioural factors that may also affect reproductive outcome (United States Congress, 1985). These factors may vary across nations and cultures, and by labour profile.

Standard-setting

Phoon (1983) suggested that the establishment of "suitable" standards should now be a top priority concern in the occupational health field. The form occupational health standards should take and their flexibility and adaptability across countries are widely debated subjects in developing countries (Christiani et al., 1990). Michaels et al. (1985) reported that in Latin America "few health standards are applied to limit work-place exposures; in most of the region's countries, the standard-setting process is either just beginning or has not yet begun. In those nations where standards regulating work practices or toxic exposure do exist, the standards are often not enforced, either for political or economic reasons or because of a lack of trained inspectors." In China a range of performance standards has been developed but they are not yet enforced and serve only as guidelines (Quinn et al., 1987). This appears to be the case in the majority of developing countries.

Standards are often modelled on those in industrialized countries and are generally not adjusted to take account of differences in such factors as climate, nutritional status, genetic predisposition, work schedules, and exposure levels (Rossiter & El Batawi, 1987; Michaels et al., 1985; Phoon, 1983). "Few developing countries have the resources to undertake the toxicologic and epidemiologic studies that serve as the necessary basis for exposure standards. Furthermore, local standard-setting processes are easily influenced by powerful economic interests" (Michaels et al., 1985).

Many countries, particularly in Africa, are just beginning to diversify their industrial sectors, hitherto confined to mining operations and agricultural processing. They face enormous obstacles in developing appropriate standards and monitoring and regulatory procedures. Research in Rwanda—a small nation with a high population density, where industrialization is proceeding at a slow pace—is already overwhelmed by the health concerns of basic industries. The country lacks the administrative and/or financial resources to develop regulatory standards or systems and must rely heavily on outside support (Blanc, 1984).

The development of appropriate and flexible international or regional standards is often recommended where governments are unable to devise their own (Michaels et al., 1985). These standards could reduce confusion over definitions of hazards and improve the transferability of technology and information (Ashford, 1985). In the future, transnational corporations operating in developing countries might be required to conform to the standards of their home country, as is proposed in a draft code prepared by the United Nations Centre on Transnational Corporations (UNCTC, 1990).

Many policy-making bodies are beginning to improve their institutional capacity to address important occupational health and safety issues. "In Egypt, Malaysia, the Philippines, and Thailand, there are top-level coordinating mechanisms between the respective government ministries with responsibilities in occupational health" (Phoon, 1983). Through the actions of the ILO, UNEP, WHO, regional bodies, and medical associations, there has been a great increase in intergovernmental exchanges on matters of, and guidelines for, occupational health and safety (El Batawi, 1981). Recently the ILO produced and disseminated a code of practice entitled *Safety, health and working conditions in the transfer of technology to developing countries* (1988). There seem to have been no studies evaluating the effectiveness of such cooperative efforts in reducing occupational hazards and/or improving workers' health.

The crucial role of labour unions in encouraging standard-setting and the enforcement of regulations in major industrial enterprises has been documented in several occupational health reviews, for countries ranging from South Africa to Brazil (Myers & Macun, 1989; Michaels et al., 1985; Castleman & Navarro, 1987; Asogwa, 1987). However, as noted in the technical discussions on intersectoral action for health held on the occasion of the Thirty-ninth World Health Assembly (WHO, 1986), workers in the informal sector, who face the greatest occupational risks, are unorganized and unlikely to benefit from policy changes resulting from union activities. There is, however, at least one encouraging exception: the Self-employed Women's Association in Ahmedabad, India, has achieved some reduction in health risks through the provision of safety gear and the improvement of working conditions by organizing a health team, educating women workers, and lobbying policy-makers. The health interests of the workers concerned were among the issues explored in the recent report of the Indian National Commission on Self-employed Women and Women in the Informal Sector (1988).

Training

The literature on occupational health in developing countries emphasizes the inadequate training provided in occupational safety and medicine for medical personnel, industrial inspectors, and workers (Shahnavaz, 1987; Nogueira, 1987; Phoon & Ong, 1985; Christiani et al., 1990). It is apparent that, in many countries, training in occupational health is not a priority for either the industrial or the health sector. Financing, manpower, technology, and educational material are all in short supply. In addition, many occupational health professionals have been trained in industrialized countries and may not be oriented to the principal occupational diseases and accidents in their home countries. Informal sector employers and small-scale industries are particularly likely to lack the resources and information needed to develop adequate supervision and training in the area of occupational health and safety (Michaels et al., 1985). In many countries, general practitioners may be on hand in industry, but not those trained in industrial medicine (Asogwa, 1987).

Progress has been made, however, in some countries which have responded to industrial growth by creating occupational health institutes focusing on important industries, such as mining and oil (El Batawi, 1981). For example, Cuba, Nicaragua, and Venezuela have developed impressive institutional support for occupational health training (Michaels et al., 1985). In Brazil, the Ministry of Labour has established an active institute for occupational safety and health, namely Fundacentro, which provides training in industrial medicine. Between 1973 and 1984, 15 000 professional health workers received training there (Nogueira, 1987). In South Africa, the labour unions have assumed a major role in informing trainers of workers' needs and in helping to determine regulatory and legislative needs (Myers & Macun, 1989). Occupational health specialists consider that health training for workers' representatives is necessary, given the limited training capacity of governments, but warn that such training will be effective only if it is accompanied by more appropriate regulations concerning the workplace (Michaels et al., 1985; El Batawi, 1981).

A guide entitled *Low-cost ways of improving working conditions: 100 examples from Asia*, produced by the ILO (Kogi et al., 1988), offers small-scale industries practical suggestions on improving the design of workstations, handling materials, housekeeping and storage, job content, and work schedules. The authors argue that small industry could use the methods recommended to reduce the costs, in terms of compensation and lost productivity, associated with occupational accidents and diseases. Unfortunately, the literature does not include an adequate analysis of the scale of such costs in developing countries. There is little information on small-scale enterprises. Because many of these are not registered, a majority of the accidents occurring in industries in the informal sector go unreported and the victims receive no compensation. As a result, it is difficult to estimate the savings effected by improving working conditions. It may nevertheless be necessary to document such savings in order to provide the economic incentive for owners of small enterprises to respond to recommendations for improvements. Case-studies of industries in the informal sector might provide useful information for governments on how to provide training in workplace design and encourage improvements in workplaces, making them economically attractive to employers in the informal sector.

Control of air and water pollution

In the past decade, the availability of data on air pollution levels in major cities has increased, although the monitoring of urban air pollution in developing countries is still in its infancy and only rough estimates are available. The Global Environmental Monitoring System (GEMS), operated jointly by WHO and UNEP, has made a significant contribution to monitoring efforts. The central activity of the GEMS programme is the measurement of sulfur dioxide levels and concentrations of suspended particulate matter in a range of cities throughout the world, selected on the basis of climate, population size, geography, and industrial base. The programme warns that its estimates are not precise enough to permit national or municipal assessments of pollution hazards and their effects on health in developing countries.

According to a GEMS estimate (WHO/UNEP, 1987), 70% of populations in the urban areas tested were living with annual average air quality conditions which were "unacceptable". Some of the probable health effects of such poor conditions are shown in Table 2. The GEMS study, however, concluded that the number of areas in which air quality is improving is greater than the number in which it is growing worse. The study did not involve any evaluation of the

Table 2. Effects of major air pollutants on health

Pollutant	Guideline values ($\mu g/m^3$ of air)		Effects of exposure
	Annual mean	98th percentile[a]	
sulfur dioxide (SO_2)	40–60	100–150	exacerbation of respiratory illness from short-term exposures increased prevalence of respiratory symptoms, including chronic bronchitis from long-term exposures
suspended particulate matter (SPM)			same as for SO_2
black smoke	40–60	100–150	combined exposure to SO_2 and SPM may have pulmonary effects
total suspended particulate matter	60–90	150–230	
lead	0.5–1	—	blood enzyme changes anaemia hyperactivity and neurobehavioural effects
nitrogen dioxide			
1 hour	400	—	effects on lung function in asthmatics from short-term exposures
24 hours	—	150	
carbon monoxide			
15 minutes	100[b]	—	reduced oxygen-carrying capacity of blood
1 hour	30[b]	—	
30 minutes	—	60[b]	
8 hours	—	10[b]	
carboxyhaemoglobin		2.5–3%	

Source: WHO/UNEP, 1989.

[a] The 98th percentile value is the concentration exceeded by fewer than 2% of the daily averages or on fewer than 7 days a year.

[b] All the values for carbon monoxide are in mg/m^3 of air.

factors contributing to this improvement or of the effectiveness of pollution control measures in developing countries.

For want of the necessary technology, infrastructure, and financial resources, it may be many years before an adequate assessment is available of the contribution made by industry to pollution-related health problems in developing countries. Little epidemiological evidence is available as yet, even in industrialized countries, from which one can predict the long-term health consequences of air pollution by industry, although important respiratory problems have been associated with high levels of ozone and carbon dioxide, and with total suspended particulate concentrations, in large urban areas in both developed and developing countries. For example, in a recent study in Mexico City, Jauregui (1987) found that there was a strong relation between the increasing incidence of acute respiratory illnesses and rising pollution levels. The highest rates of illness were observed in the industrial districts and areas where, as a result of topographical factors, pollution was concentrated. In these areas, morbidity increased substantially in the dry winter months when dust levels were 2–3 times greater than during wet periods. To respond to such pollution hazards, Mexico City has recently instituted limited restrictions on vehicle use, but has not introduced measures to reduce emissions of industrial pollutants significantly, even though they are among the main sources of pollution.

To enable pollution control efforts to be directed at the most highly polluted areas and the vulnerable groups most at risk of illness from exposure to high levels of pollution, Smith (1988) advocated an increased use of total exposure assessment (TEA) techniques which can help identify "the concentration of pollutants in the air, the duration of exposure, and the number of people exposed". Smith advocated the application of stringent air pollution standards in areas with a high population density and less stringent standards in industrial districts away from population centres. However, from preliminary TEA findings, it appears that improvements in household air quality are more readily achievable and more likely to reduce overall exposure levels in developing countries than reductions in industrial or vehicular emissions. (The health problems associated with household fuel are discussed in Chapter 5.)

Because so little is known about air pollution in developing countries, the World Bank and WHO have initiated a joint study "to identify what is common and what is location-specific to the air pollution problems in selected cities in the developing world; to establish better relationships between emissions of air pollution, air quality, human exposures and their effects on human health and the environment; to evaluate cost-effective alternative technical options to meet acceptable air quality standards, and to identify the regulatory structure, the corresponding macro-economic and sectoral measures and institutions needed to create incentives which would lead to lower pollution levels. Based on the results of the study the two institutions expect to define guidelines for acceptable levels of air pollution which can realistically be complied with under conditions of accelerated economic growth" (World Bank/WHO, 1989). Case-study findings from the cities of Ankara, Beijing, Mexico City, and Shanghai will be compared.

Industrial waste produced in developing countries is often released into, or near, lakes and streams that are untreated sources of water for large populations (Cairncross & Feachem, 1983). The risks to local inhabitants may be greater and more immediate than in industrialized countries where water is treated prior to being made available for drinking, cooking, and washing. The reliance of many people in developing countries on fishing in such polluted sources is also much greater. Heavy metals, thermal pollution, synthetic organic compounds, and pesticides have all been associated with the accidental killing of fish (Palange & Zavala, 1987). In Malaysia severe industrial pollution is produced by agro-based industries from which there are particularly heavy discharges of metal. The killing of fish by these discharges can result in loss of employment for fishermen, higher consumer prices, and reduced sources of protein (Rajeandran & Reich, 1981).

Heavy discharge of effluents from agricultural processing plants are likely to be seasonal and are especially hazardous if they occur in periods when water levels are low (Cairncross & Feachem, 1983). Toxic effluents from chemical and dye production and plating wastes are common hazards, as are heavy metal wastes from mines and factories. Since few developing countries include assessments of environmental impact in the licensing requirements for industry, the prediction of health effects is particularly problematic for industries using new chemicals or processes that are unfamiliar to government regulatory authorities.

Control of industrial pollution of water can be achieved through a variety of on-site treatments, or through municipal wastewater treatment systems, if these are available and safe (Lee, 1985). In 1987, the World Bank released a technical paper on water pollution control which provides guidelines for planners on the development of control projects (Palange & Zavala, 1987). This paper includes some background material on the sources and effects of pollution and control options, but is mainly concerned with legal, institutional, economic, and financial issues.

Some authorities in developing countries have begun imposing fines and penalties when pollution abatement objectives are not met by industry. However, the penalties tend not to be harsh and are applied infrequently and irregularly. In addition, regulations generally target new industries and have not been very effective in reducing the acute and long-term hazards associated with existing industrial facilities (see Findley, 1988). Evaluations are not yet available of the effectiveness of market mechanisms, such as pollution charges levied according to the type and quantity of pollutant produced, and other measures used to influence pollution control and improve waste disposal practices in developing countries. Lee & Lim (1983) noted that few developing countries imposed taxes on environmental pollution. They warned that market distortions, such as tariffs, prevent the efficient application of effluent charges in most developing countries. Analyses of the effectiveness of current approaches would be helpful in the future design and implementation of pollution monitoring and control programmes. An assessment of government efforts to improve access to technical information on industrial processes, inputs, and outputs is also needed if the likely sources of pollutant emissions are to be identified. So that they may institute feasible pollution charges or allocate pollution rights, developing countries will need to improve data-gathering, monitoring, and planning systems (Leonard, 1985). Increased access to low-cost pollution control equipment and technologies is needed in order to encourage pollution abatement. The ability of such measures to reduce the health problems associated with pollution is a subject for future research.

Management of hazardous wastes

Research on the health risks of toxic chemical wastes is still in its early stages, even in industrialized countries. A review of research on the public health aspects of such waste disposal sites in the USA came to the following conclusion: "Although studies of the health of populations in the vicinity of disposal sites have found only inconclusive evidence thus far implicating exposure to toxic wastes in the occurrence of disease, the following adverse health effects have been suggested: (*a*) decreased weight at birth, (*b*) increase in the frequency of congenital malformations and abortions, and (*c*) increase in the occurrence of certain forms of cancer. Further study will be required, however, to confirm the validity of these effects and to determine whether other risks may exist" (Upton et al., 1989).

The quantification and classification of industrial and hazardous wastes have been limited by problems of definition and inadequate data collection (Tolentino, 1988; Yankowitz, 1988; UNEP, 1987).

Developing countries can rarely coordinate the monitoring and regulation of hazardous waste production, transport, and disposal effectively. In some countries, no regulations on the subject have been put into force. For example, as of 1985, Mexico still had no regulations governing disposal of hazardous waste, despite the generation of an estimated 16.5 million tonnes of such waste per year (Leonard, 1986). Even where government-directed disposal programmes are developed, the health risks can still be substantial.

Open burning can create air pollution resulting in respiratory problems; sequestered disposal sites may provide opportunities for contamination of groundwater and soil; and waste may be leaked into waters used for irrigation or household use, compounding the health risks associated with the programmes (Leonard, 1986).

Cairncross & Feachem (1983) recommended that responsibility for the management and enforcement of measures related to hazardous waste be given to one national body, such as a water resource authority, that could develop flexible standards. In addition, as primary measures for the control of hazardous wastes at the production and processing stages, they recommended the registration of plants using hazardous and toxic substances and prior approval for discharge of effluents.

WHO and UNEP have developed proposals for international guidelines on the "cradle-to-grave" control of hazardous waste, including agreement on a common definition of the problem and the development of adequate model standards (WHO, 1985). WHO and UNEP indicate that simple methods still need to be developed for analysing the health effects of the transport and disposal of wastes. They recommend that governments play a bigger part in controlling the unintended adverse consequences of industrial development through the application of effective economic incentives and disincentives. The World Bank, UNEP, and WHO have sponsored case-studies on the management of hazardous wastes in developing countries, including Brazil, Malaysia, Mexico, Republic of Korea, and Thailand (World Bank/UNEP/WHO, 1987). On the basis of such case-studies, the three international organizations have jointly produced a detailed three-volume manual on the safe disposal of hazardous wastes in developing countries (World Bank/UNEP/WHO, 1989). This manual provides a framework for the evaluation of disposal options, information on the classification of wastes, an analysis of effects on the environment, advice on the planning and implementation of management programmes, and a review of the relevant political and institutional issues.

INFORM, a US-based environmental research organization, has proposed that state governments in the USA establish a hierarchy for waste management practices: (1) reduction in waste production, (2) recycling, (3) destruction, and (4) disposal (Underwood, 1988). This hierarchical approach could help improve waste management in developing countries as well. INFORM's research findings suggest that industrialized nations rely too heavily on pollution control rather than reduced production. The reasons for this appear to be "more institutional than technical, legal or economic".

A similar shift in priorities in the control of hazardous wastes is advocated for developing countries. Activities can be stimulated by improving reporting requirements, introducing waste audits, and providing economic incentives for waste reduction (Underwood, 1988). Given the difficulty of preventing health risks when destroying or disposing of hazardous wastes, this approach may be the most effective in preventing adverse effects on health.

UNEP, WHO, and other organizations are co-sponsoring training programmes in a number of countries to increase understanding by government regulatory authorities of the environmental and health risks posed by hazardous wastes, the policy levers available for the control of waste production, and management strategies appropriate to local circumstances, including the siting and development of safe landfills (UNEP, 1988). After the Bhopal disaster, stiff legislation was enacted in India to strengthen the government's power to regulate the handling of hazardous substances from manufacturing and transport to use and disposal. However, as in most developing countries, the funds and infrastructure needed to enforce this legislation are lacking (Rosencranz, 1988). Further analysis of the nature of local institutional obstacles to effective management may prove useful for future planning.

Regulatory changes may inadvertently make it harder to monitor the transport and disposal of wastes. Leonard (1986) reported that "a major concern among the newly industrializing nations is that the substantial tightening of requirements concerning hazardous wastes may be creating perverse incentives for private entrepreneurs to dispose of them in more surreptitious ways". Attempts by foreign producers, or their contractors, to offer large fees to governments in developing countries for the disposal of hazardous wastes have been widely documented (Castleman & Navarro, 1987; Leonard, 1986). Public criticism of such proposals has led to the rejection of numerous offers, although not all agreements concluded with governments in this connection have been made public. A string of countries have instituted notification requirements. Others, including the members of the Economic Community of West African States, have developed legislation making it a criminal offence to facilitate the dumping of hazardous wastes (*South,* 1988).

National health authorities can assist in devising appropriate waste policies, in evaluating the management of hazardous wastes, and in furnishing information for international negotiations on the transport and disposal of wastes. In Costa Rica, the Ministry of Health was responsible for the refusal of a request for permission to dump chemical wastes in the port of Limon (Leonard, 1986). The Minister of Health of Guinea-Bissau has objected to proposed contracts with European waste-carriers and advocated a stronger role for health ministries in setting proposals concerning waste disposal (*South*, 1988). The capacity of health authorities to assume this responsibility needs to be assessed.

Conclusion

The above review of the literature on industrial policies and health and safety shows that the links between the two have not been adequately investigated, although concern is growing about the effects of industrial development on health. The literature on industrial policies, occupational health, and environmental health does not give adequate attention to the links between health problems and policies for industrial promotion, including regulation and enforcement. Few studies have attempted to differentiate the health risks attributable to industrial policies from those caused independently by industrial decision-making, industrial action, or community behaviour. Also lacking are analyses of the process of industrial planning to find answers to such questions as: Who are the key actors in this process? What role do health authorities play in assessing the potential risks from industrial initiatives? How do health concerns figure in assessments of effects on the environment or evaluations of industrial projects?

This type of analysis may uncover important associations between policy choices and ill-health. Major policies, such as those affecting industrial specialization and the ownership and location of industries may be modified to reduce health risks and environmental hazards. Methodological advances and policy-centred case-studies could increase the ability of governments and industrial officials to design effective programmes of prevention and control.

The research reviewed here suggests that, in many cases, it is the poor who are most vulnerable to the health hazards associated with industrial development. The economic benefits of industrial activity are not necessarily experienced by those who have endured accidents, disease, or displacement. Future research on the health consequences of specific policies might focus on groups known to be vulnerable and issues of equity. Particularly weak in the literature is the analysis of policies relating to production in small industries, whether in the formal, informal, or agricultural sector, and their repercussions on the health of workers and the larger community. There are few empirical studies on the health risks associated with export processing zones that mainly employ women.

The indirect effects of industrial policies on the short- and long-term well-being of communities where industry is developing are even more difficult to assess and less well documented. The health consequences of shifting markets, resettlement, population migration, and social or ecological disruption have not been adequately explored. Further epidemiological analysis is needed to confirm the wide range of health problems associated with air and water pollution in developing countries; it is also needed by those devising strategies for pollution control and accident prevention.

There are considerable institutional, financial, and political obstacles to effective action by governments to regulate industry and promote the health of workers and communities. Nevertheless, from this review of the literature it does appear that some progress has been made in the improvement of standards and guidelines relating to industrial health, industrial safety, and the environment. In many developing countries, government policy-makers and industrial decision-makers are becoming more responsive in their planning to the concerns of workers, communities, and health authorities. Attention must now be paid to improving the contribution of governments to assessments of early risk and implications for health, to predictions of the distribution of costs and benefits, and to training, monitoring and enforcement activities, with special reference to industrial zones and regions targeted for rapid development. As part of the policy evaluation process, the health benefits of industrial development policies need to be weighed against the costs.

References

Asogwa, S. E. (1987) Prevention of accidents and injuries in developing countries. *Ergonomics,* **30**(2): 370–386.

Ashford, N. A. (1985) Policy issues in technology transfer. In: Ives, J. H., ed. *The export of hazard: transnational corporations and environmental control issues.* Boston, Routledge & Kegan Paul.

Ashworth, A. & Feachem, R. G. (1985) Interventions for the control of diarrhoeal diseases in young children: prevention of low birth weight. *Bulletin of the World Health Organization,* **63**: 165–184.

Beneria, L. & Roldan, M. (1987) *The crossroads of class and gender.* Chicago, University of Chicago Press.

Berman, D. M. (1986) Asbestos and health in the Third World: the case of Brazil. *International journal of health services,* **16**(2): 253–263.

Blanc, P. (1984) Environmental health and development in a developing country: Rwanda, a case study. *Journal of public health policy,* **5**: 271–288.

Burra, N. (1988) Exploitation of children in Jaipur gem industry. II. Health hazards of gem polishing. *Economic and political weekly,* **23**(4): 131–138.

Cairncross, S. & Feachem, R. G. (1983) *Environmental health engineering in the tropics*. Chichester, John Wiley & Sons.
Castleman, B. I. (1985) The double standard in industrial hazards. In: Ives, J. H., ed. *The export of hazard: transnational corporations and environmental control issues*. Boston, Routledge & Kegan Paul.
Castleman, B. I. (1987) Workplace health standards and multinational corporations in developing countries. In: Pearson, C. S., ed. *Multinational corporations, environment and the Third World*. Durham, Duke University Press.
Castleman, B. I. & Navarro, V. (1987) International mobility of hazardous products, industries and wastes. *International journal of health services*, 17(4): 617–633.
Christiani, D. C. (1984) Occupational health in the People's Republic of China. *American journal of public health*, 74(1): 58–64.
Christiani, D. C. et al. (1990) Occupational health in developing countries: review of the research needs. *American journal of industrial medicine*, **17**: 393–401.
de Rosen, L. (1987) Improving the working environment. *UNEP industry and environment*, **10**(3): 12–18.
Durvasula, R. S. (1988) *The development of occupational health services in India: issues of inequity and problems of regulation*. Boston, Takemi Program in International Health, Harvard School of Public Health (Research Paper No. 21).
El Batawi, M. A. (1981) Special problems of occupational health in the developing countries. In: Schilling, R. S. F., ed. *Occupational health practice*, 2nd ed. London, Butterworths.
El Batawi, M. A. & Husbumrer C. (1987) Epidemiological approach to planning and development of occupational health services at a national level. *International journal of epidemiology*, **16**(2): 288–292.
Feachem, R. G. (1986) Preventing diarrhoea: what are the policy options?. *Health policy and planning*, 1(2):109–117.
Findley, R. W. (1988) Pollution control in Brazil. *Ecology law quarterly*, 15(1): 1–68.
Forssman, S. (1981) Health in small industries. *World health*, November, pp. 20–22.
Fuentes, A. & Ehrenreich, B. (1984) *Women in the global factory*. Boston, South End Press.
Galenson, A. (1984) *Investment incentives for industry: some guidelines for developing countries*. Washington, DC, World Bank (Staff Working Paper No. 669).
Gladwin, T. N. (1987) A case study of the Bhopal tragedy. In: Pearson, C. S., ed. *Multinational corporations, environment and the Third World*, Durham, Duke University Press.
Hamer, A. (1985) Urbanization patterns in the Third World, *Finance and development*, 22(1): 39–42.
Hovell, M. F. et al. (1988) Occupational health risks for Mexican women: the case of the Maquiladora along the Mexican-United States border.

International journal of health services, **18**(4): 617–627.

Huddle, N. & Reich, M. (1987) *Island of dreams: environmental crisis in Japan*. Rochester, VT, Schenkman Books.

Indian National Commission on Self-Employed Women and Women in the Informal Sector (1988) *Commission report: Shramshakti*. New Delhi.

ILO (1988) *Safety, health and working conditions in the transfer of technology to developing countries*. Geneva, International Labour Office.

ILO/UN Centre on Transnational Corporations (1985) *Women workers in multinational enterprises in developing countries*. Geneva, International Labour Office.

Jasanoff, S. (1985) Remedies against hazardous exports: compensation, products liability and criminal sanctions. In: Ives, J. H., ed. *The export of hazard: transnational corporations and environmental control issues*. Boston, Routledge & Kegan Paul.

Jauregui, E. (1987) Incidence of respiratory illness and air pollution levels in Mexico City. *Climate and human health: world climate programme applications*. Geneva, World Meteorological Organization.

Kamuzora, P. (1986) Redefining occupational health for Tanzania. *Review of African political economy*, **36**: 30–34.

Kogi, K. et al. (1988) *Low-cost ways of improving working conditions: 100 examples from Asia*. Geneva, International Labour Office.

Kramer, M. S. (1987) Determinants of low birth weight: methodological assessment and meta-analysis. *Bulletin of the World Health Organization*, **65**(5): 663–737.

Lave, L. B. & Seskin E. P. (1977) *Air pollution and human health*. Baltimore, Johns Hopkins University Press.

Ledec, G. & Goodland, R. (1984) *The role of environmental management in sustainable economic development*. Paper presented at the annual meeting of the International Association of Impact Assessment.

Lee, J. K. & Lim, G. C. (1983) Environmental policies in developing countries: a case of international movements of polluting industries. *Journal of development economics*, **13**: 159–173.

Leonard, H. J. (1985) Confronting industrial pollution in rapidly industrializing countries: myths, pitfalls, and opportunities. *Ecology law quarterly*, **12**: 779–816.

Leonard, H. J. (1986) Hazardous wastes: the crisis spreads. *Asian national development*, April, pp. 33–42.

Leonard, H. J. (1988) *Pollution and the struggle for the world product*. Cambridge, Cambridge University Press.

Lepkowski, W. (1987) The disaster at Bhopal—chemical safety in the Third World. In: Pearson, C. S., ed. *Multinational corporations, environment, and the Third World*. Durham, Duke University Press.

Levenstein, C. & Eller, S. W. (1985) Exporting hazardous industries: "For example" is not proof. In: Ives, J. H., ed. *The export of hazard: transnational corporations and environmental control issues*. Boston, Routledge & Kegan Paul.

Michaels, D. et al. (1985) Economic development and occupational health in Latin America: new directions for public health in less developed countries. *American journal of public health,* **85**(5): 536–542.

Myers, J. E. & Macun, I. (1989) The sociological context of occupational health in South Africa. *American journal of public health,* **79**(2): 216–224.

Naidu, U. S. & Kapadia, K. R., ed. (1985) *Child labour and health: problems and prospects.* Bombay, Tata Institute of Social Sciences.

Nogueira, D. P. (1987) Prevention of accidents and injuries in Brazil. *Ergonomics,* **30**(2): 387–393.

Noweir, M. H. (1986) Occupational health in developing countries with special reference to Egypt. *American journal of industrial medicine,* **9**: 125–141.

Packard, R. M. (1989) Industrial production, health and disease in sub-Saharan Africa. *Social science and medicine,* **28**(5): 475–496.

Palange, R. C. & Zavala, A. (1987) *Water pollution control: guidelines for project planning and financing.* Washington, DC, World Bank.

Pearson, C. S. (1987) Environmental standards, industrial relocation, and pollution havens. In: Pearson, C. S., ed. *Multinational corporations, environment, and the Third World.* Durham, Duke University Press.

Phillips, M. A. et al. (1987) *Options for diarrhoea control: the cost and cost-effectiveness of selected interventions for the prevention of diarrhoea.* London, London School of Hygiene and Tropical Medicine (Evaluation and Planning Centre for Health Care (EPC) Publication No. 13).

Phoon, W. O. (1983) Occupational health in developing countries: a simple case of neglect. *World health forum,* **4**: 340–343.

Phoon, W. O. & Ong, C. N., ed. (1985) *Occupational health in developing countries in Asia.* Tokyo, Southeast Asian Medical Information Centre.

Pimenta, J. C. P. (1987) Multinational corporations and industrial pollution control in São Paulo, Brazil. In: Pearson, C. S., ed. *Multinational corporations, environment, and the Third World.* Durham, Duke University Press.

Pitt, D. C. (1985) Child labour and health. In: Naidu, U. S. & Kapadia, K. R., ed. *Child labor and health: problems and prospects.* Bombay, Tata Institute of Social Sciences.

Quinn, M. M. et al. (1987). Modernization and trends in occupational health and safety in the People's Republic of China, 1981–1986. *American journal of industrial medicine,* **12**: 499–506.

Rajeandran & Reich, M. R. (1981) Environmental health in Malaysia. *The bulletin of the atomic scientists,* **37**(4): 30–35.

Rosencranz, A. (1988) Bhopal, transnational corporations, and hazardous technologies. *Ambio,* **17**(5): 336–341.

Rossiter, C. & El Batawi, M.A. (1987) The working environment. *UNEP industry and environment,* **10**: 3–11.

Shah, P. M., ed. (1985) *Child labour: a threat to health and development.* Geneva, Defence for Children International.

Shahnavaz, H. (1987) Workplace injuries in the developing countries. *Ergonomics,* **30**(2): 397–404.

Singh, A. M. & Kelles-Viitanen, A., ed. (1987) *Invisible hands: women in home-based production*. New Delhi, Sage Publications.

Smith, K. R. (1988) Air pollution: assessing total exposure in developing countries. *Environment,* **30**(10): 16–20, 28–34.

South (1988) The dumping grounds. August, pp. 37–41.

Sun, Y. (1989) Export processing zones in China. Buji: a case study. *Economic and political weekly,* **24**(7): 355–365.

Thomas, V. (1985) Evaluating pollution control: the case of São Paulo, Brazil. *Journal of development economics,* **19**: 133–146.

Thomas, V. (1981) *Pollution control in São Paulo, Brazil: costs, benefits and effects on industrial location*. Washington, DC, World Bank (Staff Working Paper No. 501).

Tolentino, A. S. (1988) Hazardous waste management in the ASEAN: an emerging regime. *UNEP industry and environment,* **11**(1): 28–29.

Tower, E. (1986) Industrial policy in less developed countries. *Contemporary policy issues,* **4**(1): 23–35.

Townroe, P. M. (1983) *Location factors in the decentralization of industry: a survey of metropolitan São Paulo, Brazil*. Washington, DC, World Bank.

UNCTC (1990) *The New Code Environment*. New York, United Nations Centre on Transnational Corporations (Current Studies, Series A, No. 16).

Underwood, J.D. (1988) Managing hazardous waste is not enough. *UNEP industry and environment,* **11** (1): 29–31.

UNEP (1987) *Environmental data report*. New York, United Nations Environment Programme.

UNEP (1980) *Guidelines for assessing industrial environmental criteria for siting of industry*. New York, United Nations Environment Programme.

UNEP (1988). The United Nations environment programme activities in hazardous waste management. *UNEP industry and environment,* **11**(1): 32–37.

USAID (1980) *Environmental design considerations for rural development projects*. Washington, DC, Harza Engineering Company for United States Agency for International Development.

United States Congress (1985) Office of Technology Assessment. *Reproductive health hazards in the workplace*. Washington, DC, US Government Printing Office (OTA-BA-266).

Upton, A. C. et al. (1989) Public health aspects of toxic chemical disposal sites. *Annual review of public health,* **10**: 1–25.

Van Esterik, P. & Greiner, T. (1981) Breastfeeding and women's work: constraints and opportunities. *Studies in family planning,* **12**(4): 182–195.

Vining, D. R. (1985) The growth of core regions in the Third World. *Scientific American,* **252**(4): 42–49.

Warr, P. G. (1989) Export processing zones: the economics of enclave manufacturing. *Research observer,* **4**(1):65–88.

Whittemore, A.S. (1981) Air pollution and respiratory disease. *Annual review of public health,* 2: 397–429.

WHO (1986) *Intersectoral action for health.* Geneva, World Health Organization.

WHO (1988) *Training manual on research and action methodologies and techniques concerning the health of working children.* Unpublished WHO document, MCH 88.2.

WHO/FAO/UNEP (1985) Panel of Experts on Environmental Management for Vector Control (PEEM). *The environmental impact of population resettlement and its effect on vector-borne diseases* (technical discussion at the Fifth Meeting of PEEM, October 1985). Unpublished WHO document, VBC 85.5.

WHO/UNEP (1987) *Global pollution and health: results of health-related environmental monitoring.* Unpublished WHO document.

WHO/UNEP (1989) Monitoring the global environment: an assessment of urban air quality. *Environment,* 31(8): 6–13, 26–37.

Wintemute, G. J. (1986) Injury mortality and socioeconomic development: an exploratory analysis. *International journal of epidemiology,* 15(4): 540–543.

Wolman, A. (1980) Health and the environment. *Bulletin of the Pan American Health Organization,* 14(1): 6–14.

World Bank (1987) *Environment, growth, and development.* Washington, DC, World Bank and IFC Development Commitee.

World Bank/WHO (1989) *Comparative air pollution study proposal: case study of air pollution in Ankara.* Washington, DC, World Bank.

World Bank/UNEP/WHO (1987) *Hazardous waste management in the Third World.* Washington, DC, World Bank.

World Bank/UNEP/WHO (1989) *The safe disposal of hazardous wastes: the special needs and problems of developing countries.* Washington, DC, World Bank.

Yankowitz, H. (1988) Identifying, classifying and describing hazardous wastes. *UNEP industry and environment,* 11(1): pp. 3–10.

CHAPTER 5

Energy policies

Developing countries have begun substituting commercial fuels—mainly coal and petroleum products—for traditional biofuels and charcoal. However, this movement up the "energy ladder" has been affected by continual fluctuations in the price of imported petroleum, and most countries remain heavily dependent on biofuels. Accompanying this transition from one type of fuel to another has been a rapid increase in the overall demand for energy, creating strains on the economy and the environment. Industrial and domestic consumption of commercial fuels has greatly increased pollution, and the development of hydropower has brought with it additional hazards. A rising urban demand for wood fuel, in both the industrial and domestic sectors, has contributed to deforestation and its attendant problems in many parts of the world. For poor rural and urban households, the increasing scarcity of wood fuel has meant reduced fuel consumption, or a return to the use of animal wastes and other less efficient and more highly polluting fuels. These emerging "energy crises" signal a need for more coherent and effective planning in the energy sector.

As fuel scarcity, fluctuations in fuel prices, and environmental problems increase, governments are seeking ways of increasing their influence over energy use. Measures under consideration include identifying alternative energy sources, encouraging appropriate fuel pricing and substitution, increasing access to technology for the enhancement of fuel efficiency, and improving environmental planning in major energy projects. But the impact of government decisions on the supply, demand, or use of energy in developing countries remains poorly understood. Under these circumstances, health does not appear to be a priority concern for those developing and evaluating energy policy. Nevertheless, there is a growing body of literature on the health risks associated with energy extraction, generation, and use. Less widely examined have been the effects of energy policies on the health problems of rural or urban communities, and it is not easy to find examples of direct policy measures that effectively lessen energy-related risks to health.

This chapter deals with: the effects on health of fuel use in the home and associated efforts to control indoor air pollution; the effects of fuel scarcity on the health of households; the effects of fuel pricing, substitution, and subsidies; control of pollution from industrial energy sources; and the health hazards presented by hydroelectric power projects. Its review of these subjects suggests that the absence, rather than the presence, of explicit development policies in the energy sector may have the most pronounced effect on the health and welfare of the poor.

Important matters that are not explored here include the injuries resulting from accidents involving kerosene or other petroleum-related fuels in the workplace and in the home; health risks associated with the expanding petrochemical industry; the effects on nutrition of reduced crop yields linked to soil depletion and deforestation due to energy extraction; the hazards presented by fossil fuels and nuclear energy; and the long-term risks associated with the greenhouse effect and acid rain.

Indoor air pollution and domestic fuel use

A recent publication, *Biofuels, air pollution and health: a global review* (Smith, 1987), examines a vast array of scientific analyses covering such aspects of biofuel use as indoor air pollution levels, human exposure levels, and implications for health. This volume, which appears to be the most in-depth and up-to-date survey of the links between domestic fuel use and health conditions, includes a bibliography with over 400 references. It concludes that, while more evidence is required to determine the strength of the association between health problems and the combustion of biofuels indoors in developing countries, greater attention to the policy implications of this association is warranted.

The severity of the health risks presented by indoor air pollution depends on the length and level of exposure to pollutants emitted by fires using wood, animal dung, scrub plants, or crop residues as fuel. Women and children in developing countries who spend hours in unventilated structures exposed to smoke from cooking stoves face the greatest health risks from indoor air pollution. It is estimated that approximately half the world's households cook daily with biofuels. Used mainly for cooking, these fuels account for over one-third of all energy consumed in developing countries (Smith, 1987). In some countries, biofuels also provide the energy for space-heating. On the basis of the limited data available, it is estimated that exposure to pollutants is 60 times greater in indoor environments in the rural areas of developing countries than in the urban areas of developed countries (Smith, 1988). Overall daily exposures are estimated to be 20 times greater in developing than in developed nations (Pandey et al., 1989). The UNEP/WHO Global Environmental Monitoring System (GEMS) is pursuing research on indoor air pollution through its Human Exposure Assessment Location Project. Recent studies in Kenya (WHO/UNEP, 1987) and the Gambia (WHO/UNEP, 1988) have reported an association between high levels of respirable suspended particulate matter and the combustion of wood and crop residue fuels.

Research over the last decade has linked the use of unprocessed biomass fuel to the incidence of respiratory infections. Studies of indoor air pollution and respiratory function in developing countries are difficult to compare owing to the variability of the sampling methods employed and inadequacies of design. Nevertheless, evidence from retrospective case–control and cohort studies in China, India, Nepal, Nigeria, Papua New Guinea, South Africa, and other countries suggests that there is a strong relationship between indoor combustion of biofuels, high concentrations of airborne particulate matter, and acute respiratory infections (see Smith, 1987 for references). The most serious problems include bronchitis and pneumonia in children, and chronic bronchitis and other chronic pulmonary disease in adults, particularly women (Smith, 1987; Stansfield, 1987; Pio, 1986; Malik, 1985.) In addition, although a causal relationship has not been confirmed, indoor air pollution is seen as a potentially important risk factor for low birth weight (Kramer, 1987).

The health risks presented by indoor air pollution may be greatly increased by associated environmental health risks. For example, the inhalation of fuel smoke, when combined with cigarette smoking or passive smoking, appears to increase the risk of respiratory problems and low birth weight still further (Smith, 1988). With the increasing incidence of smoking in many developing countries, efforts to reduce this combination of risks are becoming all the more urgent.

The flow-chart in Fig. 3 summarizes the relationships between domestic and community behaviour, fuel combustion, and health effects, and can serve as a basis for policy discussions in the energy and environmental health sectors in developing countries. As the chart suggests, there is an important relationship between the effects of indoor air pollution on health and the underlying health and

Fig. 3. Framework for the study of the place of biofuel combustion in the rural life of developing countries.[a]

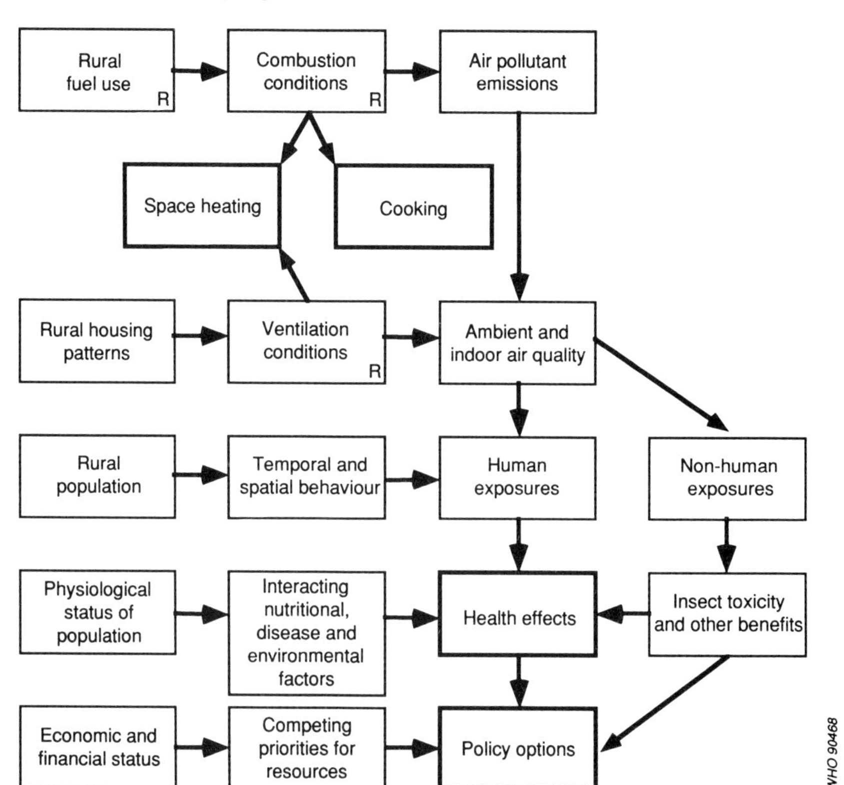

Source: Smith, 1987. Reproduced by permission of the publisher.
[a] The letter R denotes areas where technical remedies are most readily available.

nutritional status of the population. Additional geographically specific research is required to provide the basis for appropriate policy measures targeting those most at risk.

Biofuels are not the only energy source making a substantial contribution to indoor air pollution and ill-health in developing countries. In Shanghai, China, a 12-year follow-up study was conducted on 957 males who participated in a screening programme for coronary heart disease and stroke (Zhang et al., 1988). The study found that, in addition to the expected risk factors for stroke, including diastolic blood pressure, age, and cigarette smoking, there was an independent risk factor, namely exposure to coal fumes. The authors of the study considered this finding important, since coal fumes are a major source of indoor air pollution in China. In Shanghai, for example, 50% of households use coal for fuel. It was concluded that methods to improve air quality, such as the elimination of coal-burning stoves, could contribute to a reduction in mortality from stroke. A recently completed study in Beijing found a significant association between elevated sulfur dioxide levels from domestic coal use and decreased pulmonary function, particularly in densely populated areas (Xu et al., 1989). Given China's continued primary reliance on coal for its energy needs, the substitution of other fuels for domestic use is unlikely. Reduction of the health risks through energy conservation and pollution control may be the only feasible short-term strategy. "Smokeless" coal stoves that release their fumes outside the dwelling are being developed in China, Mexico, and other countries.

Control of indoor air pollution

Methods for the measurement of indoor air pollution concentrations and exposure levels, and for the estimation of the associated health risks, are still inadequate, even in industrialized countries (Sexton & Repetto, 1982). Contradictory findings and a lack of conclusive evidence have slowed the process of translating research conclusions into policy recommendations. Furthermore, the regulation of indoor air quality is particularly difficult. In the USA, for example, while outdoor air is looked on as a public concern, indoor air is not. In an analysis of indoor air pollution and public policy issues, Sexton & Repetto (1982) asserted that the effectiveness of public policy interventions would depend on their ability to inform and improve private choices regarding use of energy and consumer products, smoking, and other behaviour. They recommended focusing on low-cost measures, such as public information compaigns, warning devices, product-testing, and product-labelling.

These measures would not be effective in reducing the primary sources of indoor air pollution in developing countries. Poor consumers in these countries are faced with economic pressures and fuel shortages that prevent them from responding to information-based approaches alone. But the overall policy objectives proposed by Sexton & Repetto—to inform and improve private choices—may be appropriate. National energy policies in developing countries could help improve access to low-cost safe fuels and cooking methods, along with appropriate consumer education. Nevertheless, this would present a major challenge, since the communities most at risk also appear to be the most difficult to reach.

One measure would be to improve access to cleaner processed fuels. For reasons of safety and efficiency, commercial fuels such as kerosene and liquid petroleum gas, as well as charcoal, ought to be given preference over biofuels for domestic consumers in developing countries. However, these fuels are often priced beyond the reach of low-income populations (see the discussion of fuel pricing on pp. 107–110). Only as incomes rise is a transition to processed fuels apparent. Nevertheless, a switch to these fuels does not necessarily ensure safety, as they have proved hazardous in the absence of proper safety education or appropriate appliances. Domestic accidents involving kerosene have been widely reported, particularly in poor urban communities, and emissions of kerosene smoke have been linked to heart and lung problems. Charcoal may be safer than many biofuels in the long run, but charcoal combustion carries a risk of acute carbon monoxide poisoning (Smith, 1987). The environmental problems associated with charcoal production (see below) may also have adverse consequences for health in some rural areas. Thus, improvements in domestic ventilation and education on safe fuel use may be critical for the success of any effort to promote alternatives to biofuels.

Nevertheless, as affordable processed fuels are unlikely to become available to rural communities and fuel scarcity is a growing problem, the safe and efficient use of biofuels will remain a priority concern of policy-makers (Smith, 1987). Indoor air pollution analysts (Pandey et al., 1988) advocate measures to reduce indoor air pollution as part of energy, housing, and health programmes addressing a variety of risk factors. Programmes for improving biofuel cooking-stoves are seen by Smith (1987) as one of the principal steps towards the reduction of indoor air pollution in both rural and urban areas. The expansion of programmes to improve fuel efficiency and safety is discussed below, together with some of the problems involved. But first there is a discussion of another energy-related source of health risks for poor households: fuel scarcity.

Fuel scarcity

It is estimated that more than one thousand million people live in woodless rural areas in developing countries; 230 million urban residents are also affected by fuel poverty. More than 100 million people are estimated to lack the minimum requirements for domestic fuels for cooking and lighting (FAO, 1983). The response of planners in the energy sector to the root causes of fuel scarcity, such as deforestation, has so far been limited, and the needs of rural consumers have been particularly neglected (Wilbanks, 1987).

The growing problem of deforestation in developing countries has been closely linked to fuel poverty and its consequences. The available evidence suggests that deforestation is largely attributable to the commercialization of wood fuel and charcoal for urban markets and not to rural consumption patterns, as previously believed (Tinker, 1987). Teplitz-Sembitzky & Schramm (1989) concluded that "it is the overall framework of development rather than energy demand of the residential sector which is at the heart of the problem". They identified industrial activities, unplanned settlements, agricultural expansion, urbanization, and population growth as more significant factors in deforestation than fuel demand. Pearson & Stevens (1989) suggested that deforestation was also related to the relative value of various options for land use. The production of wood fuel may be a less profitable enterprise than the clearance of forests for cultivation or other purposes. Government-determined stumpage fees and licence fees for wood harvesting from publicly managed forests are generally set too low, encouraging rapid forest clearance and generating revenues that cover only a small portion of forest replacement costs (Repetto, 1989).

In urban areas, cooking fuels, such as wood, are generally available only from commercial sources (Leach & Gowen, 1987). Deforestation occurs rapidly on the routes leading out of urban areas in many developing countries as the urban demand for wood fuel grows (see, for example, Bowonder et al., 1986). As nearby sources of energy are depleted, wood and charcoal are transported from greater distances and larger rural areas are affected (Leach & Gowen, 1987). Thus, in many countries, the increasing urban demand for wood fuel has contributed to deforestation, encouraged the commercialization of rural fuel supplies, and increased the fuel poverty of rural consumers. The scarcity of fuel resources for poor urban and rural households can have a variety of impacts on health status, as discussed below.

Fuel-gathering: a time-consuming activity

Often attributed to deforestation, increases in the time required for the collection of wood fuel in rural areas have been documented in time-allocation studies in a range of developing countries. Since women and children in most developing countries have primary responsibility for gathering firewood, its scarcity has increased the demand made on women's time, affecting their families and their own welfare by leaving them less time for preparing food, making extra income, working in the fields, looking after children, and consulting health services (Cecelski, 1984; Tinker, 1987; Stone & Molnar, 1986; Pearce, 1985; Berio, 1984). Recent research in south India has shown that women, even in rural areas, purchase firewood to save the time they would have spent gathering it, thus freeing themselves for other tasks, but also reducing their disposable income (Tinker, 1987). The effects on health and nutrition of this shift in spending were not explored, but the research suggests that efforts to reduce the time spent gathering wood may also have indirect negative effects on a household's health and nutritional status. Given the variable quality and comparability of time-allocation studies, additional country-specific data are required in order to explore these hypotheses adequately. If they hold true, policy options can be suggested to reduce energy-related time constraints. Pearson & Stevens (1984) included the opportunity cost of labour used in gathering firewood in their "augmented energy balance matrix", which is designed to facilitate the analysis, on a national level, of traditional and commercial practices relating to the supply and consumption of energy. This may be one approach to the task of ensuring that household-level concerns are taken into account in national energy policies.

Given the effects of energy expenditure on people's health and nutrition, a reduction in the energy requirements for fuel-gathering and cooking might be one means of reducing health risks for women and children in rural areas. Policies which increase access to fuel, time-saving techniques, and prepared food, such as bread, can help reduce energy expenditure and improve nutritional status, resistance to disease, and birth weights (McGuire & Popkin, 1989; Tinker, 1987; Berio, 1984; Batliwala, 1981). On the basis of research on energy supply and consumption, as well as time-allocation studies, Batliwala (1981) estimated that the cost, in calories, of the collection of fuel and water, cooking, and other domestic chores represented nearly one-third of the daily energy expenditure of women in India. Batliwala suggested that an increased availability of appropriate technology and alternative fuel sources could make an important contribution to the reduction of human energy expenditure, but warned that additional research on time allocation and energy consumption was required to assess the impact it would have on health. McGuire & Popkin (1989) suggested that development programmes should be designed to increase women's productivity in the household and motivate them to allocate more time to rest and child care, thus helping to improve the health and nutritional status of their families. Energy programmes seeking to promote efficiency and safety in the use of fuel in the home might incorporate these objectives and coordinate their activities with those of other programmes relating to family health and nutrition.

Changing cooking practices

The increasing scarcity of wood fuel has led to changes in cooking habits that have been shown to have an adverse effect on food intake, thus potentially harming the health and nutritional status of families. Reductions in the consumption of cooked foods, associated with the scarcity of affordable cooking fuels, have been recorded in Nepal and Rwanda, and a reduced intake of staple foods has been noted in Guatemala, Mexico, and Somalia (Cecelski, 1987; Leach, 1984). Studies of the allocation of resources within households have shown that women and children in particular may suffer deprivation as a result of food scarcity or loss of income (Bennett, 1988; Piwoz & Viteri, 1985; Carloni, 1981; Chen et al., 1981).

Even when the time spent in obtaining fuel is reduced, other time constraints may limit the efficient use of fuel in cooking. Research in Burkina Faso, India, Java, and Nepal has shown that the activity on which women spend most time every day is the processing and preparation of food, and that they may use several stoves at once in an attempt to save time (Tinker, 1987). In many urban areas, poor women are increasingly turning to food preparation as a money-making activity, thus spending more time cooking and increasing fuel consumption (Tinker, 1987). With the resultant intensification of indoor air pollution, the health risks to their families may be increased. For other women, the availability of prepared foods may reduce the time spent on cooking, but can increase overall food costs. In some countries, such as Kenya, a number of different fuels and cooking-stoves are used, depending on season, time of day, and the food being cooked (Hyman, 1987). Additional comparative studies are required to ascertain the prevalence of the various cooking practices, related pollution levels, and associated effects on health. Such research would be of value to policy-makers seeking to improve fuel conservation, safety, and household welfare.

Improvement of cooking-stoves

Programmes for the improvement of cooking-stoves with the aim of reducing the demand for wood fuels, or alleviating fuel poverty through a more efficient use of fuel in the home, have been adopted in pilot areas in developing countries with mixed success. Many of these programmes have failed to produce changes in cooking practices and fuel efficiency for a number of reasons. Initially, they were rarely integrated into rural development schemes or primary health care activities, did not stimulate sufficient interest or compliance, and were difficult to sustain (Smith, 1987; Gill, 1987). In addition, they have also proved ineffective in reaching women and in adapting to local social and cultural conditions (Tinker, 1987; Carloni, 1987).

Technological changes to improve fuel efficiency or safety in domestic cooking often require a significant time investment. Tinker (1987) asserted that stove improvement programmes had generally failed to take into consideration the "inelasticity" of rural women's time, which restricts their ability to consider technological alternatives, or to invest time in learning about and installing new stoves, or in adapting to new cooking practices. Tinker concluded that the dissemination of new stoves was likely to be more successful in urban than in rural areas, because of the more favourable climate for behavioural change and new technology that exists in the towns.

Most programmes to disseminate improved cooking techniques promote stove models or appliance adjustments that increase fuel efficiency, but these rarely incorporate smoke-reduction features that can alleviate indoor air pollution (Smith, 1987). The *Household energy handbook* produced by the World Bank (Leach & Gowen, 1987) suggests that the dissemination of fuel-efficient stoves can improve hygiene, health, and child safety. However, both Smith (1987) and Tinker (1987) argued that improvements in health do not necessarily follow stove improvement programmes, since the technology advocated may involve neither improvement of ventilation nor smoke reduction. Reduced smoke, reduced fuel usage, and ease of use must all be viewed as objectives in the design of stoves and in ensuring their effective dissemination and use so that it may be possible to achieve a marked reduction in pollution levels.

Manibog (1984) listed six primary conditions for effective and sustainable stove improvement programmes that would result in a more efficient use of fuel. While they contain no direct reference to improving fuel safety and health, they are all probably necessary in order to achieve these objectives: "(1) active participation by women (stove users), artisans, and the marketing and disseminating (e.g., extension) workers in developing or adapting a stove design; (2) proof that long-run market, production, delivery, and maintenance systems exist or can be established; (3) establishment of training programs for local artisans or extension workers; (4) development of strong financial support for a strategy to market the chosen stoves and appliances based on comprehensive acceptance surveys and, possibly, incentive pricing systems to stimulate early adoption of the new technology; (5) continued support for research and monitoring of stove development; and (6) market conditions which allow competitive models to be developed and reach the market."

In the past decade, progress has been made in improving the design, adaptability, and acceptability of fuel-efficient cooking-stoves, although much still needs to be done to make them safer. In Kenya, charcoal stoves are used by approximately 83% of urban households and 17% of rural households, and labourers in Nairobi may spend up to 25% of their income on charcoal (Hyman, 1987). A joint effort by international agencies such as USAID and UNICEF and local nongovernmental organizations has succeeded in developing low-cost, low-technology, fuel-efficient stoves which have been distributed to several hundred thousand Kenyan homes through programmes in the informal and private sectors (Hyman, 1987; World Resources Institute/International Institute for Environment and Development, 1987).

In Burkina Faso, self-help programmes have been initiated which offer training in the construction of highly fuel-efficient "three stone stoves" from locally available materials, for rural households that cannot afford to pay upfront costs for new stoves (World Resources Institute/International Institute for Environment and Development, 1987). The World Bank/UNEP Energy Sector Management Assistance Programme is also supporting locally organized stove improvement programmes in a number of countries.

The objectives of programmes to improve cooking-stoves may be counteracted by government fuel policies. In some countries government price controls on charcoal have worked against efforts to promote fuel conservation (Hyman, 1987). Coordination of the objectives of fuel pricing and fuel conservation programmes may be essential in order to achieve gains in fuel efficiency and reduce fuel poverty. In addition, the improvement of stove safety must be given a more prominent place in these programmes if health improvements are to be achieved. Cost-effectiveness analyses in specific countries may provide programmes with useful guidance on how to achieve the greatest gains in terms of fuel efficiency and pollution reduction.

Even when fuel efficiency and safety have been achieved, households may still suffer the health consequences of fuel poverty, if fuel remains scarce. Households headed by women are likely to be at highest risk, owing to the many demands on the women's time, their low social status in many countries, and financial constraints. Several studies have found that women are often denied, or do not seek, access to wood fuel produced in cash-crop plantations (Spears & Winterbottom, 1985). The coordination of afforestation schemes with rural energy programmes, such as stove distribution and education, may help improve patterns of fuel supply and consumption for the poorest rural households. Nevertheless, Pearson & Stevens (1989) argued that, despite better targeting in stove improvement programmes in recent years, "it is not difficult to demonstrate that, on a variety of working assumptions, the impact of woodstoves on wood use, and even more, on deforestation, is likely to be small and possibly expensive, especially in relation to other policy instruments". Other energy policies that may help reduce fuel poverty and its impact on health are described below.

Fuel pricing, substitution, and subsidies

Pearson & Stevens (1989) argued that fuel scarcity was largely the result of faulty pricing: "Wood is priced 'too low' and/or commercial energy is priced 'too high'." High importation and transport costs can result in commercial fuel prices that are a strain on the incomes of poor households. Although wood fuel is a depletable resource, the user costs or opportunity costs, if it is gathered by the consumer rather than purchased, are not taken into account in the price. Costs relating to the environmental aspects of wood-burning are also not considered in determining the price. In addition, the time and energy involved in gathering fuel are expended by women, who rarely control household spending. Thus, issues of both efficiency and equity are raised by decisions on fuel pricing.

In urban areas, lack of access to direct sources of domestic fuel means that low-income populations are required to purchase traditional or commercial fuels which are often of low quality and contain high concentrations of pollutants. Like their rural counterparts, low-income urban residents are faced with the health risks posed by cooking and heating with unprocessed fuels in crowded and poorly ventilated dwellings. Even in rural areas, acute fuel scarcity can increase demand and prices in local wood fuel markets, placing a heavier burden on household budgets.

The potential impact of fuel costs on household purchasing power and health status is likely to be similar to those of food pricing and housing costs, as discussed in chapters 2 and 6. As energy prices increase, the quality of the fuels accessible to low-income populations decreases while the proportion of household resources spent on energy needs increases. This may leave less money for food and potentially lower the nutritional status of the members of the household. As noted above, disparities in the allocation of food within a household may put women and children at particularly high risk. Further investigation is warranted to uncover the cumulative effect of increasing fuel, food, and housing costs on health in both urban and rural households.

Given the cost of petroleum products, wood fuel is usually cheaper than any commercial fuel substitute (Teplitz-Sembitzky & Schramm, 1989). Conflicting evidence, however, is provided by research in India, where Bowonder et al. (1986) found that forest depletion had reached such proportions in some areas that wood fuel costs had increased at a much faster rate than the consumer price index. As a result, low-income populations had to spend more of their income on wood fuel or, alternatively, turn to kerosene, which was comparatively lower in price. Because of fluctuations in the prices of kerosene, coal, and liquid petroleum, wood fuel remains the most affordable option overall and increases in the price pose a major challenge to poor households. There are a number of exceptions, however: in Indonesia, kerosene has replaced wood fuel because of the shortage of wood and, in China, coal has supplanted wood as the primary source of household energy, even in rural areas (Sathaye & Meyers, 1987). High wood fuel prices also appear to be responsible for an increase in the illegal extraction and sale of wood fuel by the rural poor, which may increase income in the short run but will reduce agricultural productivity and fuel resources in the long run.

The scarcity of wood fuel has made substitution of other fuels a necessity. Pearson & Stevens (1989) listed five possible responses to the situation: (1) to switch to "unsafe wood", which further contributes to soil erosion, silting, flooding, and desertification; (2) to switch to less efficient biofuels ("trade down"), such as animal and vegetable residues; (3) to switch to commercial fuels ("move up-market"), such as oil, coal, gas and electricity; (4) to improve the availability of new wood supplies through reforestation, and improve fuel efficiency through changes in fuel appliances; and (5) to do nothing, thus accepting fuel scarcity and creating more fuel poverty. The potential health effects of each of these choices have been discussed above, but the short- and long-term health and welfare trade-offs have not been carefully assessed. A comparison between them could help government efforts to encourage appropriate changes in fuel pricing and in household decision-making. Reforestation and fuel substitution strategies would be more effective if accompanied by community initiatives promoting income-generation or employment, since household poverty remains at the root of many of the interactions between fuel use and health.

Government pricing policy

To make it easier for poor households to afford fuel, governments have often sought to influence fuel prices. In some countries, price controls have been imposed, but the resulting reductions in the supply of commercial fuel may offset the benefits of the lower prices. Pachauri & Pachauri (1985) suggested that the "transition away" from oil, which occurred in the early 1980s in many developing countries, was principally due to hikes in oil prices and not to any deliberate policy measures imposed on commercial or domestic consumers. They contended that in most countries there was a marked absence of effective policy-making with regard to energy. To improve this situation they recommended increased training in energy planning and in energy sector analysis in developing countries. Other energy analysts agree about the lack of integrated energy planning, particularly as regards inclusion of the traditional fuel market, and consider that progress has been hampered by institutional weaknesses (Wilbanks, 1987; Pearson & Stevens, 1984). In developing countries, energy policy has been most rigorous in restricting private operations in the oil industry and controlling prices, although many governments are beginning to loosen controls in order to increase the role of market competition in regulating oil prices. Where this type of energy-pricing strategy is employed, trade-offs between macroeconomic efficiency and equity are inevitable (Krapels, 1988).

Bowonder et al. (1986) have offered the following policy options for maintaining wood-fuel resources in India: distribution of kerosene to low-income populations; the introduction of high-efficiency kerosene cooking-stoves; and improved access to liquid petroleum gas for commercial users. Pearson & Stevens (1989) advocated a number of broader policy options to reduce fuel poverty, including the use of targeted subsidies to improve access to more expensive commercial fuels and efficient cooking and heating appliances. They also called for measures to secure a steady supply of alternative fuels, estimation of anticipated costs and benefits, and assessment of the administrative and political feasibility of the alternative policy options proposed. They warned, however, that policies aimed at the energy sector alone would not alleviate fuel poverty, and pointed to the need for programmes to supplement the income of poor households.

Even if alternative fuels are made available at lower costs, consumers may not be aware of their fuel options. In India, for example, it was found that "for historical reasons poorer sections of the population believe that fuelwood is the cheapest source of fuel"

(Bowonder et al., 1986). It is uncertain whether similar perceptions exist in other countries, but this finding suggests that public education is required on the prices of alternative fuels, as well as on the hazards of using wood as fuel, to reduce undue reliance on wood and improve household safety.

Fuel subsidies and taxes

Fuel subsidies have been implemented in various countries to improve the accessibility of low-income populations to commercial fuels and to improve fuel markets. However, the successful targeting of fuel subsidy programmes to the poor has proved elusive. Research has demonstrated that the benefits of kerosene subsidies have often leaked to producers and to moderate- and high-income groups (Pearson & Stevens, 1989). Nevertheless, the World Bank/UNEP Energy Sector Management Assistance Programme (ESMAP) has reported that reductions in fuel subsidies may have extremely harmful consequences for low-income groups (World Bank, 1988b). The removal of fuel subsidies has been one feature of the government response to recent economic crises in many countries. The effects on nutrition may be similar to those observed in connection with the reduction of food subsidy programmes during periods of adjustment (see Chapter 2). However, empirical research is lacking on the health effects of fuel subsidy programmes or their curtailment.

Research in Thailand on the effects of fuel taxes on income found that kerosene taxes had a slightly regressive effect, which was likely to be particularly marked in rural households that relied on kerosene as their primary cooking fuel (Hughes, 1983). This effect could be offset by reducing export taxes on rice or other agricultural commodities, thereby favouring rural producers and providing an incentive for greater allocative efficiency in the energy and agricultural sectors. An assessment of the costs and benefits to health of generating revenue through fuel taxes might be warranted. However, it is unlikely that direct associations would be easily identified, and even more unlikely that tax policies would be altered as a result of evidence of adverse repercussions on health. An analysis of the level of sales taxes across a variety of sectors might provide a more powerful indication of how the health of poor populations could be affected. In such an assessment, it would also be important to examine budgetary allocations of tax revenues: are these revenues used to support health services or energy supply programmes?

Control of pollution from industrial energy sources

The results of the few studies that have examined concentrations of air pollutants in cities in developing countries reveal an inverse relationship between income levels and urban air pollution. The poorer cities experience a "risk overlap"—pollution due to the domestic use of solid fuels, including wood and coal, is combined with highly concentrated emissions of pollutants from industrial undertakings and vehicles (Smith, 1988). Effective strategies for pollution control thus depend on cooperation between energy planners, industrial officials, and environmental and health authorities.

In developing countries, industry accounts for 25–40% of total national energy consumption and consumes the bulk of commercial fuels (Anandalingam, 1985). Emissions from power stations using high-sulfur coal and oil are considered to be making an increasingly large contribution to hazardous levels of air pollution in the urban areas of developing countries. In addition to the long-term environmental degradation that is predicted as a result of acid deposition, these emissions may contribute to respiratory problems and related ailments among populations living close to their sources. However, few studies attribute existing health problems in urban areas directly to these sources. In 1979, the United Nations Economic Commission for Europe released a report containing a checklist of environmental and technological concerns relating to a broad range of energy-producing facilities, but it did not cover probable risks to health (United Nations Economic Commission for Europe, 1979). UNEP has begun efforts to assess emissions from fossil fuels, nuclear fission, and hydroelectric power plants and their effects on health (UNEP, 1985a, 1985b). UNEP is also conducting cost-benefit analyses of various approaches to emission control. In China, where coal combustion is the principal source of atmospheric pollution, three low-cost control measures are being promoted: reduction of ash and sulfur content in coal preparation, improved dust collection, and use of coal briquets (Zhao & Sun, 1986).

Energy extraction, particularly coal-mining, has long been associated with serious occupational health hazards in developing countries. While programmes to prevent accidents and occupational diseases have met with some success, the air and water pollutants released by the expanding mining activities in many countries, such as Malaysia and Papua New Guinea, are an increasing source of concern. There is little epidemiological evidence of the long-term effects of mining dust, toxic metallic effluents, and other pollutants on the health of communities living near mining operations (Down &

Stocks, 1977). Although predictions of health effects remain tenuous, regulatory measures to control pollution in densely settled areas have been adopted by some developing nations. The speed with which energy sources are being uncovered and exploited may, however, prove too great for countries to be able to prevent adverse effects on the environment. These industries are among the principal earners of foreign exchange for many developing economies. Policy-makers are therefore faced with difficult trade-offs between health, the environment, and the economy in their decisions on land use and energy planning. These decisions are made all the more difficult by scientific uncertainty regarding both short- and long-term risks.

As noted in the previous chapter, total exposure assessments have suggested that, in many developing countries, short-term policy interventions may be more effective if they concentrate on reducing domestic rather than industrial pollution. The immediate risks associated with domestic pollution may be more extreme, and the populations affected, greater. It will take more substantial policy interventions over the long term to reduce fossil-fuel emissions from industry as well as vehicular pollution in countries where the commercial use of energy is rising rapidly (Smith, 1988). Total exposure assessment (TEA) techniques may be helpful in setting priorities and identifying targets for pollution control in developing countries. However, before policy decisions can be made, these techniques must be subjected to more rigorous testing (Smith, 1988). The financial requirements of the TEA approach may prove to be a major obstacle. Many countries continue to lack the resources and manpower to perform basic pollution measurements. Nevertheless, countries such as the United Republic of Tanzania are investigating ways of improving government monitoring of energy emissions and of strengthening incentives and legal authority for pollution control (Nkoniki & Lushiku, 1988).

In some countries where petroleum prices are rising, industries are substituting coal for oil, which is likely to create new health hazards and problems of acid rain. Other industrial substitutes, such as charcoal and geothermal energy, can also create serious health and environmental problems. Less hazardous energy sources, such as biofuel gasifiers, bagasse, wind, and solar energy, are also being investigated in developing countries by agencies dealing with energy and the environment. Despite the major obstacles to be overcome in assessing effects on health and improving pollution control, measures are being taken to increase fuel conservation by both government and industry in developing countries. ESMAP is supporting efforts to reduce hazardous emissions. Nevertheless, energy analysts consider that fuel subsidies to stimulate industrial growth will have to be curtailed to ensure that fuel conservation becomes a priority (Anandalingam, 1985).

Many analysts also advocate the coordination of bioenergy programmes with overall agricultural policies (Ramsey, 1985; Bhatia, 1985). There is concern, for example, at the fact that the concentration of energy production in urban and industrial areas has created serious problems for the agricultural sector, which has become dependent on imported oil. With the aim of improving agricultural productivity and the nutritional status of rural consumers, Lewis (1984) has called for a policy of decentralization that will promote local sources of energy.

Health risks presented by hydroelectric power programmes

Development of hydropower is a priority for many developing countries. The World Bank's Energy Department has predicted that "hydropower will continue to play a significant role in developing power programs, accounting for 43% of electricity production by 1995" (World Bank, 1984). Most dams constructed primarily for generation of hydropower have been large, with significant associated health and environmental risks that have rarely been adequately addressed.

Chapter 3, on agricultural policies, reviewed the literature on the health consequences of irrigation schemes. The myriad health problems associated with hydroelectric or multipurpose dam projects are similar in nature to those resulting from other schemes for the development of water resources. Hunter et al. (1982) have examined the relationships involved in great depth.

As irrigation projects are usually in densely populated areas, the health hazards associated with them tend to be more severe than those associated with hydroelectric dams, which are located in more isolated regions (Hunter et al., 1982). Hydroelectric projects can still have adverse effects on local communities, as a result of increases in vector-borne diseases and the involuntary resettlement of people from areas that have had to be flooded. Precisely because hydropower projects are not commonly viewed as community development schemes, as are many irrigation programmes, poor planning for resettlement and rehabilitation can result in a variety of health and welfare problems (World Bank, 1989).

A number of water-related diseases have been causally linked with the creation of reservoirs and the resettlement of populations when dams are built. Of greatest concern, and most widely documented, have been significant increases in the transmission of schistosomiasis and malaria, particularly where water impoundments provide breeding-sites for the vectors. The spread of onchocerciasis in populations living near dam spillways and downstream has also been reported. Project feasibility studies will have to include better assessments of health risks, if disease prevention and control programmes are to be effectively implemented at an early stage of the project.

Dam projects can also result in lowered nutritional status, as highly productive fields are flooded, thereby reducing both commercial and subsistence food production. Downstream fishing may also be restricted by the prevention of fish migration and changes in water quality. However, given proper planning, these effects can be offset by reservoir fishing and increased agricultural yields in new fields provided by irrigation in multipurpose dam projects (World Bank, 1989).

The absence of proper housing, screening, and health services for dam construction workers and for resettled populations can increase disease transmission, as can the interaction of local communities and migrants hoping to benefit from the development of the area. Cultural disruption and social alienation of uprooted communities have also commonly occurred with resettlement (see Goldsmith & Hildyard, 1986; Cernea, 1988a; Nachowitz, 1988; Ablasser, 1987; World Bank, 1988a, 1989). Goodland & Post (1989) suggested that health, housing, and agricultural programmes for the resettled populations should be integrated into regional development schemes, in order to reduce the health and welfare problems associated with resettlement.

The World Bank has instituted policies on involuntary resettlement and rehabilitation for the major water resource development and agricultural projects it supports (Cernea, 1988b; Escudero, 1988). These policies aim at ensuring that the economic resources, services, and living standards of the resettled communities are at least equivalent to those they enjoyed prior to resettlement. Since the World Bank finances only 3%, and plays a role in approximately 10%, of all hydroelectric projects in developing countries (Goodland & Post, 1989), it is unclear how great an effect this policy will have in reducing the health problems of resettled populations. Even when the policies are adopted, their objectives may not be achieved. For example, it has been reported that, in the Narmada Valley water development projects in India, the World Bank's resettlement policies have been adopted by the local authorities and widely publicized, but that significant problems exist in connection with their implementation, particularly as regards ensuring land transfers (Sarangi & Billorey, 1988). Without land, the development of adequate food resources for household nutrition is likely to be seriously restricted. Greater attention to the effective implementation of resettlement policies is thus of crucial importance in hydroelectric projects.

The health problems associated with hydroelectric projects may also be connected with accompanying industrial development, as well as with changes in agriculture, housing, services, and water resource management. Industries sometimes develop alongside hydroelectric facilities to take advantage of the energy resources available. The pollutants these industries release into waterways present a threat to health and the environment (Goodland, 1985). "As major investments, dams can have large impacts on regional development and induce growth of new population centers and industrial activity. The cumulative effects of such projects may be substantially different from the effects of individual projects" (Dixon et al., 1989). In a number of countries, consortia of industrial enterprises have been formed to ensure the full use of the power produced by major hydroelectric projects. Goldsmith & Hildyard (1986) contended that this could lead to the uncontrolled growth of hazardous industries in proximity to hydropower sources. However, there appears to have been no further research to confirm this conclusion.

Delays in the planning and implementation of major water development projects can also create health-related problems for nearby populations. In India, surveys for the programme for the development of water resources in the Narmada Basin were initiated forty years ago, but work on the numerous dam projects involved began only recently. Owing to the area's uncertain future, housing assistance, services, and new roads were not provided to local residents during the long planning period. Unemployment has remained high, with little new investment in the area (*Economic and political weekly*, 1988). Thus, health and nutritional problems may have been exacerbated by the delay in implementing the development plans. Assessments of the health, welfare, and economic repercussions of such delays might prove useful in preventing the deprivation of communities in future projects.

Injuries, deaths, and displacement due to dam bursts, or to safety and operational problems with dams, have occurred in countries throughout the world. Such accidents and problems have been linked to poor design, the use of low-quality materials, and errors of construction. UNEP recently reviewed existing data on the consequences of dam bursts in the last two decades (UNEP, 1987a). Of the 11 major dam bursts from 1965 to 1985 reported in the UNEP document, 7 were in developing countries. Of the deaths resulting from these accidents, 99% occurred in the developing countries. While a number of the accidents were due to earthquakes, mud-slides, and floods, UNEP noted that structural weaknesses and construction flaws were major contributory factors.

The spread of small hydroelectric projects in many developing countries is expected to increase the number of communities at risk (Hunter et al., 1982). The proliferation of water impoundments, environmental disruption, and construction deficiencies, as well as limited planning and resources for preventive action, are expected to contribute to increased disease transmission, higher injury rates, and related problems, despite improved planning for large-scale programmes.

While the World Bank's policies on the effects of dam projects on the environment are likely to improve planning and maintenance and reduce health risks in the projects supported by that organization, similar guidelines need to be developed for smaller-scale projects and locally supported efforts. The latter constitute the vast majority of projects under way. Rapid assessment of the health risks associated with water resource development projects has been urged, together with increased attention to the trade-offs between health costs and benefits (Prost, 1987; Gratz, 1987). In the opinion of Fearnside (1988) an effort must be made to ensure that such assessments become more than formalities in the project development process. In many countries, the environmental and public health authorities lack any bargaining power in projects to develop natural resources. Some improvement in their institutional clout and authority in project planning is needed to enhance the role of health impact assessments in determining the design of such projects and their follow-up.

The principal recommendations concerning research, policy, and planning adjustments presented in Tiffen's guidelines on the incorporation of health safeguards into irrigation projects through intersectoral cooperation (1989; see also Chapter 3) also apply to hydroelectric projects. Areas where planning might be improved include: assessment of health risks in pre-feasibility studies; increased training in the appropriate assessment methods for health professionals, engineers, and contractors; the inclusion of health costs in calculations of the internal rate of return; and increased interministerial coordination as regards the preparation, design, operation, and maintenance of projects. A comparative analysis of institutional processes for the planning of hydroelectric projects, and other major initiatives for the development of water resources, could be helpful in improving the guidelines so that they can be adapted to local conditions.

Conclusion

In many countries, health risks may arise more from the absence of policy-making in the non-commercial energy sectors than from the effects of explicit policies. There is increasing evidence of the wide range of health problems associated with uncontrolled trends in energy demand, supply, and use in developing countries. These include the problems associated with indoor air pollution generated by fuel combustion; with reduced food consumption resulting from fuel poverty or the cost of commercial fuel; and with changes in the time allotted to household responsibilities, which may affect family care. There are also the health risks associated with industrial power stations, including hydropower plants; and the long-term health risks expected as a result of resource depletion and environmental degradation. The profound associations between poverty, energy choices, and health are particularly striking.

More attention now needs to be paid to the policy levers available for the reduction of immediate health risks. Some energy analysts warn, however, that attempts to deal with major environmental or development problems through policy levers in the energy sector may be inappropriate and could ultimately reduce the overall effectiveness of energy planning by diluting its objectives (see, for example, Pearson & Stevens, 1989). It may therefore be essential for health and energy authorities to develop priority strategies for tackling immediate health threats created by energy extraction and fuel use. Energy planners require more longitudinal data on trends in energy supply and consumption in order to assess appropriate targets for intervention more effectively.

Despite the increasing amount and improved quality of research on the adverse health effects of indoor air pollution due to domestic fuel use, there have been few examinations of the links between national and local energy policies, household practices, and health conditions. Progress has been made in providing access to appropriate technology for improving fuel efficiency in some areas. Similar efforts need to be made to ensure that cooking-stove designs are safe as well as efficient, and that any distribution of stoves is accompanied by education on fuel safety.

To modify fuel and stove use by a majority of the populations currently at risk in developing countries, government intervention will undoubtedly be necessary. Fuel prices have been shown to have an important effect on the choice of domestic fuel, but the effects of government pricing measures on poor consumers need to be further explored. An additional effort should be made to ensure that such measures help to reduce the fuel poverty of low-income rural and urban households. Improved targeting of fuel subsidy programmes is required, as is better analysis of the health implications of reductions in subsidies.

Progress has been made in assessing the important health risks associated with hydroelectric projects in a wide range of countries. It is evident, however, that most developing countries require an improved planning framework for hydroelectric projects, incorporating assessments of the health and social effects as well as an analysis of the effect on the environment. Owing to problems of implementation, measures to provide health services or disease control programmes during and after dam construction tend to be inadequate. More attention needs to be paid to the reduction of health risks in small-scale hydroelectric projects and to improved implementation of environmental and health measures to help resettled populations.

As a result of the overall scarcity of energy sources in most developing countries, industrial energy policies will need to develop alongside domestic energy policies, and both will need to reflect an awareness of the health risks associated with specific strategies. In the matter of supply and demand, traditional fuels have not been given adequate attention compared with that given commercial fuels. At present, most countries need better data and analyses of data, on which to base a coordinated planning strategy. The World Bank/UNEP Energy Sector Management Assistance Programme may be an appropriate model for activities at both the national and the international level. This programme operates in both the domestic and the industrial energy sector and advocates integrated energy planning and policies. More interaction between energy planners and those involved in monitoring and assessing the effects on health of indoor and outdoor pollution from energy sources would also help improve policy measures for pollution control, the reduction of risks, and health provision in rural and urban areas.

References

Ablasser, G. (1987) Issues in settlement of new lands. *Finance and development*, 24(2): 45–48.

Anandalingam, G. (1985) Energy conservation in the industrial sector of developing countries. *Energy policy*, 13(4): 335–339.

Batliwala, S. (1987) *Rural energy scarcity and nutrition: a new perspective.* Bombay, Foundation for Research in Community Health.

Bennett, L. (1988) The role of women in income production and intra-household allocation of resources as a determinant of child nutrition and health. *Food and nutrition bulletin*, **10**(3): 16–26.
Berio, A. (1984) The analysis of time allocation and activity patterns in nutrition and rural development planning. *Food and nutrition bulletin*, **6**(1): 53–68.
Bhatia, R. (1985) Energy and agriculture in developing countries. *Energy policy*, **13**(4): 330–334.
Bowonder, B. et al. (1986) Fuelwood prices in India: policy implications. *Natural resources forum*, **10**(1): 5–16.
Carloni, A. S. (1981) Sex disparities in the distribution of food within rural households. *Food and nutrition*, 7: 3–12.
Carloni, A. S. (1987) *Women in development: AID's experience, 1973–1985. Vol. 1. Synthesis paper*. Agency for International Development, Washington, DC (AID Program Evaluation No. 18).
Cecelski, E. (1987) Energy and rural women's work: crisis response and policy alternatives. *International labour review*, **126**(1): 41–64.
Cernea, M. M. (1988a) Involuntary resettlement and development. *Finance and development*, **25**(3): 44–46.
Cernea, M. M. (1988b) *Involuntary resettlement in development projects: policy guidelines for World Bank-financed projects*. Washington, DC, World Bank (Technical Paper No. 80).
Chen, L. C. et al. (1981). Sex bias in the family allocation of food and health care in rural Bangladesh. *Population and development review*, 7(1): 55–76.
Dixon, J. A. et al. (1989) *Dams and the environment: considerations in World Bank projects*. Washington, DC, World Bank (draft).
Down, C. G. & Stocks, J. (1977) *Environmental impact of mining*. London, Applied Science Publishers.
Economic and political weekly (1988) Of forests and people. **23**(25): 1264–1265.
Escudero, C. R. (1988) *Involuntary resettlement in bank-assisted projects: an introduction to legal issues*. Washington, DC, World Bank.
FAO (1983). *Fuelwood supplies in the developing countries*. Rome, Food and Agriculture Organization of the United Nations (Forestry Paper 42).
Fearnside, P. M. (1988) China's Three Gorges Dam: "fatal" project or step toward modernization?. *World development*, **16**(5): 615–630.
Gill, J. (1987) Improved stoves in developing countries. *Energy policy* **15**(2): 135–144.
Go, F. C. (1987) *Environmental impact assessment: an analysis of the methodological and substantive issues affecting human health considerations*. Geneva, World Health Organization/Monitoring and Assessment Research Centre (MARC Report No. 41).
Goldsmith, E. & Hildyard, N. (1986) *The social and environmental effects of large dams*. San Francisco, Sierra Club Books.
Goodland, R. & Post, J. (1989) *The World Bank's new policy on the environmental aspects of dam and reservoir projects*. Washington, DC, World Bank (draft).

Gratz, N. (1987) *Why risk assessment for water development projects?* Background paper for World Bank Workshop on Assessment of Human Health-Risks in Irrigation and Water Resource Development Projects, Paris.

Hughes, G. A. (1983) *The impact of fuel taxes in Thailand.* Washington, DC, World Bank (draft).

Hunter, J. M. et al. (1982) Man-made lakes and man-made diseases: towards a policy resolution. *Social science and medicine,* **16**: 1127–1145.

Hyman, E. L. (1987) The strategy of production and distribution of improved charcoal stoves in Kenya. *World development,* **15**(3): 375–386.

Kramer, M. S. (1987) Determinants of low birth weight: methodological assessment and meta-analysis. *Bulletin of the World Health Organization,* **65**(5): 663–737.

Krapels, E. N. (1988) Evolution and reform: the art of transition in energy pricing policy. *Natural resources forum,* **12**(3): 221–233.

Leach, G. & Gowen, M. (1987) *Household energy handbook: an interim guide and reference manual.* Washington, DC, World Bank (Technical Paper No. 67).

Leach, G. & Mearns, R. (1989) *Beyond the woodfuel crisis: people, land and trees in Africa.* London, Earthscan.

Lewis, C. (1984) The need for an alternative energy strategy in the agricultural economies of the Third World. *Energy,* **9**(8): 651–659.

Malik, S. K. (1985) Exposure to domestic cooking fuels and chronic bronchitis. *Indian journal of chest diseases and allied sciences,* **27**(3): 171–174.

Manibog, F. (1984) Improved cooking stoves in developing countries: problems and opportunities. *Energy,* **9**: 197–227.

McGuire, J. & Popkin, B. M. (1989) *Increasing women's resources for nutrition in developing countries.* Presentation to the United Nations Coordinating Committee's Subcommittee on Nutrition, Symposium on Women and Nutrition, New York.

Nachowitz, T. (1988) Repression in the Narmada Valley, India. *Cultural survival quarterly,* **12**(3): 23–25.

Nkonkiki, S. R. & Lushiku, E. (1988) Energy planning in Tanzania: emerging trends in planning and research. *Energy policy,* **16**(3): 280–291.

Pachauri, R. K. & Pachauri, R. (1985) Energy problems and policies in developing countries. *Energy policy,* **13**(4): 301–303.

Pandey, M. R. et al. (1989) Indoor air pollution in developing countries and acute respiratory infection in children. *Lancet,* **1**(8635): 427–429.

Pearce, D. (1985) *The major consequences of land and water mismanagement in developing countries.* Washington, DC, World Bank (draft paper for the Projects Policy Department).

Pearce, D. (1989) Energy and environment. *Energy policy,* **17**(2): 82–83.

Pearson, P. J. G. & Stevens, P. J. (1984) Integrated policies for traditional and commercial energy in developing countries. *Development policy review*, 2: 131–153.

Pearson, P. J. G. & Stevens, P. J. (1989) Fuelwood crisis and the environment: problems, policies and instruments. *Energy journal*, 17(2): 132–137.

Pio, A. (1986) Acute respiratory infections in children in developing countries: an international point of view. *Pediatric infectious disease journal*, 5(2): 179–183.

Piwoz, E. G. & Viteri, F. E. (1985) Studying health and nutrition behaviour by examining household decision-making, intra-household resource distribution, and the role of women in these processes. *Food and nutrition bulletin*, 7(4): 1–32.

Prost, A. (1987) *Critical review and case study materials*. Background paper, World Bank Workshop on Assessment of Human Health Risks in Irrigation and Water Resource Development Projects, Paris.

Ramsey, W. (1985) Biomass energy in developing countries. *Energy policy*, 13(4): 326–329.

Repetto, R. (1989) Economic incentives for sustainable production. In: Schramm, G. & Warford, J., ed., *Environmental management and economic development*, Baltimore, MD, Johns Hopkins University Press (for the World Bank).

Sarangi, S. & Billorey, R. (1988) The nightmare begins: oustees of Indira Sagar Project. *Economic and political weekly*, 23 April, pp. 829–830.

Sathaye, J. & Meyers, S. (1987) Transport and home energy use in cities of the developing countries: a review. *Energy journal*, **8**: 85–103.

Sexton, K. & Repetto, R. (1982) Indoor air pollution and public policy. *Environment international*, **8**: 5–10.

Smith, K. R. (1987) *Biofuels, air pollution, and health*. New York, Plenum Press.

Smith, K. R. (1988) Air pollution: assessing total exposure in developing countries. *Environment*, **30** (10): 16–20, 28–34.

Spears, J. & Winterbottom, R. (1985) *Tropical forestry action programme: fuelwood and social forestry*. Washington, DC, World Resources Institute (discussion draft).

Stansfield, S. K. (1987) Acute respiratory infections in the developing world: strategies for prevention, treatment and control. *Pediatric infectious disease journal*, **6**: 622–629.

Stone, A. & Molnar, A. (1986) *Issues: women and natural resource management* (with Bibliography: women and resource management in developing countries). Washington, DC, World Bank.

Teplitz-Sembitzky, W. & Schramm, G. (1989) Woodfuel resource use and environmental management. *Energy policy*, April, pp. 123–131.

Tiffen, M. (1989) *Guidelines for the incorporation of health safeguards into irrigation projects through intersectoral cooperation, with special reference to vector-borne diseases*. Unpublished WHO document VBC/89.5.

Tinker, I. (1987) The real rural energy crisis: women's time. *Energy journal*, 8 (special LDC issue): 125–146.

United Nations Economic Commission for Europe (1979) *Environment and energy: environmental aspects of energy production and use with particular reference to new technologies.* London, Pergamon Press for the United Nations.

UNEP (1985a) *Phase I. Comparative data on the emissions, residuals and health hazards of energy sources.* Paris, United Nations Environment Programme (Energy Report Series, ERS-14-85).

UNEP (1985b) *Phase II. Cost-benefit analysis of the environmental impacts of commercial energy sources and its use in emission control of energy systems.* Paris, United Nations Environment Programme (Energy Report Series, ERS-15-85).

UNEP (1987a) *Environmental data report.* Oxford, Blackwell.

UNEP (1987b) Environmental management of petrochemicals and downstream industries. *Industry and environment,* **10**(1): 1–2.

Wilbanks, T. J. (1987) Lessons from the national energy planning experience in developing countries. *Energy journal,* **8** (special LDC issue): 169–182.

World Bank (1984) *A survey of the future role of hydroelectric power in 100 developing countries.* Washington, DC (Energy Department Paper, No. 17).

World Bank (1988a) *Indonesia: the transmigration program in perspective.* Washington, DC (World Bank Country Study).

World Bank (1988b) Energy Sector Management Assistance Programme. *Annual report.* Washington, DC.

World Bank (1989) Environment Department. *The large dam controversy.* Washington, DC (draft).

WHO/UNEP (1987) Global Environmental Monitoring System, Heal Project. *Indoor air pollution study, Maragua area, Kenya.* Unpublished WHO document, WHO/PEP/87.7.

WHO/UNEP (1988) Global Environmental Monitoring System, Heal Project. *Indoor air quality in the Basse area, The Gambia.* Unpublished WHO document, WHO/PEP/88.3.

World Resources Institute/International Institute for Environment and Development (1987) *World resources 1987.* New York, Basic Books.

Xu, X. et al. (1989) *Air pollution and its effect on pulmonary function in Beijing, China.* Research paper, Takemi Program in International Health, Harvard School of Public Health, Boston.

Zhang, Z. et al. (1988) Indoor air pollution of coal fumes as a risk factor of stroke, Shanghai. *American journal of public health,* **78**(8): 975–977.

Zhao, D. & Sun, B. (1986) Atmospheric pollution from coal combustion in China. *Journal of the American Pollution Control Association,* **36**: 371–374.

CHAPTER 6

Housing policies

By the year 2000, nearly half of the population of developing countries will reside in urban areas and 50 of the world's 66 largest cities—each with more than four million inhabitants—will be in developing countries (Jensen, 1988). While, in many developing countries, major urban areas may still be relatively small, the rate of their expansion, through natural population growth and migration, is outstripping the planning and management capacity of governments. Almost half the residents of these cities live in unplanned settlements or slums without legal title to the land they occupy. In many urban areas, 70% of slum residents are in families headed by women (WHO, 1987a). Because of the rapid expansion of low-income urban populations, governments will need to provide 65% more services, including water and sanitation, by the end of the century simply in order to maintain current standards (Jensen, 1988). Improvements in the quality of services will be an even greater challenge. The reduction of ill-health among low-income urban dwellers will depend to a large extent on such improvements.

The World Bank has identified two types of urban policy: the first encompasses measures to affect migration patterns, urbanization trends, and the distribution of populations; the second is based on the management of urban problems as they arise (World Bank, 1983). The emphasis here will be on the latter, because of its direct relevance to urban housing conditions and health, but clearly the former has a profound indirect effect. A number of urban housing policies have been adopted to provide for the needs of low-income populations and to reduce the spread of illegal subdivisions and squatter settlements. Many of these strategies have an unintended impact on health and social welfare.

This chapter explores the literature on urban housing policies in the following areas: housing conditions and health; implementation of housing programmes, including clearance; public housing provision; sites-and-services programmes; upgrading of slums and squatter settlements; and standard-setting and regulation.

Important housing and health concerns not explored in these pages include: the interactions between urban employment, industrial development, housing, and health; the formal rental housing market and health conditions; land-use planning and environmental health; relocation and resettlement schemes; and water supply and sanitation programmes. This chapter concentrates on urban housing policies, because environmental health problems in rural areas are more apt to be linked to the absence of policies on housing and infrastructure development rather than to the unintended consequences of explicit policies.

Housing conditions and health

A considerable literature has developed on the links between health and housing. Most studies have incorporated concern for water, sanitation, and related infrastructure and services into their definitions of housing. A similar approach is used in this chapter, which is concerned with what may be termed the housing or home environment. Thus, the housing policies considered here are those that address the need not only for the construction of dwellings, but also for a variety of services and infrastructural elements associated with the home environment. However, there is still a lack of epidemiological evidence concerning the precise association between structural components and health conditions. It may be that policies that encourage the construction, destruction, or alteration of dwellings may have little direct effect on health conditions, but a substantial indirect effect, for example, by increasing poverty.

In 1976, WHO published a lengthy annotated bibliography on housing and health, which included epidemiological studies on the complex associations between housing, the housing environment, and health (Martin et al., 1976). This publication covered such topics as the siting, construction, and habitation of housing, water supply and sanitation, and the effects of air, water, and noise pollution. Most of the studies reviewed were based on research in the industrialized countries.

More recent analyses of housing and health in developing countries show a strong association between ill-health and both quantitative and qualitative shortcomings in water supply, food supply, and sanitation. Inadequate shelter, poor ventilation, lack of facilities for solid waste disposal, air and noise pollution and overcrowding are also likely to have negative consequences for health (Harpham et al., 1988; WHO, 1987a; Stephens et al., 1985; USAID,

1981). Table 3 presents a summary of major health problems associated with housing conditions and suggests appropriate ways of dealing with them through design. Table 4 presents estimates of the numbers of people throughout the world affected by poor housing

Table 3. Features of housing design and diseases they may help to overcome

Design feature	Diseases combated
Strong association	
*adequate supply of water	trachoma, skin infections, gastroenteric diseases
*sanitary excreta disposal	gastroenteric infections including intestinal parasites
*safe water supply	typhoid, cholera
*bathing and washing facilities	schistosomiasis, trachoma, gastroenteric and skin diseases
*means of food production	malnutrition
+control of air pollution	acute and chronic respiratory diseases and malignancies
Fairly strong association	
*ventilation of houses (where there is smoke from indoor fires)	acute and chronic respiratory diseases
control of house dust	asthma
*siting houses away from vector-breeding areas	malaria, schistosomiasis, filariasis, trypanosomiasis
+control of open fires, protection of kerosene or bottled gas	burns
*finished floors	hookworm
*screening	malaria
*wall integrity and sound house structure; hut design and location of beds and animals	Chagas disease, tick-borne relapsing fever
Some association	
*control of use of thatch material	Chagas disease
*rehabilitation of housing	psychological disorders
*+control of heat inside shelter	heat stress
adequate food storage	malnutrition
*refuse collection	Chagas disease, leishmaniasis, gastro-enteric diseases

*Problems that may be tackled through housing policies and programmes (including water and sanitation needs).
+Problems that may be tackled through energy policies and programmes (including improvement of cooking-stoves and promotion of safe fuels (see Chapter 5, Energy policies)).
Modified from Stephens et al., 1985.

Table 4. Estimates of morbidity, mortality, and disability related to housing conditions

Aspect of housing	Example of related health problem	Total global morbidity (millions)	Approximate proportion of total global morbidity related to given aspect of housing (%)	Approximate annual numbers of illnesses, deaths, and long-term disabilities related to given aspect of housing		
				illnesses (millions)	deaths (millions)	long-term disabilities (millions)
house-based parasites	Chagas disease	17	100	17	2	2
breeding of vectors (mosquitos)	malaria	100	50	50	1	—
lack of water and sanitation	child diarrhoea and poliomyelitis	1000	25	250	1	0.1
physical structure of house, cooking facilities, etc.	domestic injuries and burns	30	100	30	0.3	0.3
indoor air pollution	chronic respiratory disease	30	50	15	0.5	—
climate	heat stress, hypothermia, acute respiratory infections	—	—	—*	—*	—

construction materials	lead poisoning, lung cancer	—	—	—*	—*	—
crowding	tuberculosis	25	10	2.5	0.1	—
heating, outdoor air pollution	chronic respiratory disease	—	—	—*	—*	—
transportation	traffic accident injuries	50	10	5	0.1	0.1
food storage	salmonellosis	—	—	—*	—*	—

— = no estimate made.
* = insufficient data available, but the figures may be as high as for the other problems.
Source: WHO, 1987a.

conditions. As the figures suggest, the associations between health and housing are of varying strength, and the strength of many of them is still subject to debate. The influence of housing on malaria transmission, for example, may be exaggerated. Some of the conditions listed in this table, such as indoor air pollution, poor cooking appliances, and fuel poverty among low-income urban and rural populations, were considered in the previous chapter.

As noted by Stephens et al. (1985), although the associations between health and the housing environment are well documented, it is difficult to isolate and substantiate causal relationships. A variety of factors complicate the issue, including income, employment, and educational status. The social dynamics and behavioural patterns of urban life may further complicate the situation, by fostering exposure to particular health risks, such as sexually transmitted diseases, substance abuse, child abuse, stress-related illness, and inadequate nutritional intake due to expenditure on alcohol or luxury items rather than food (Harpham et al., 1988; WHO, 1987a; Stephens et al., 1985).

While overall health indices suggest that urban residents fare better than rural populations, the poorest urban communities may exhibit more alarming health and nutritional conditions than their rural counterparts, and disparities in the distribution of resources and services in cities are extreme (Rossi-Espagnet, 1987). Unfortunately, data on health status differentials in urban areas remain limited in many countries. Most city or municipal health data are presented in aggregate form (Rossi-Espagnet, 1987). The assessment of health conditions and their probable causes in squatter settlements and urban slums is complicated by the lack of baseline health data, the instability of populations, and the sheer growth of the communities concerned. In order to determine the scope and seriousness of urban health problems, data from a number of urban areas are required (Basta, 1982). Disaggregation and careful analysis of case studies on health and urban conditions will be required to identify policy influences.

Findings from stratified analyses of urban nutrition data in a number of cities show that the energy intake of residents of slums or squatter settlements is generally one-half to two-thirds the city average, vitamin A intake one-third to one-half the aggregate level, and the prevalence of anaemia twice as great as the citywide average, while approximately 10% of slum and settlement children suffer from severe malnutrition (Basta, 1977; see also: Kerejan & N'da, 1981; de la Luz Alvarez et al., 1979; Sigulem & Tudisco, 1980; Data Banik, 1977, 1979). Other analyses of nutrition-related health problems in urban areas include those by Popkin & Bisgrove (1988),

Viteri (1987), and Hussain & Lunven (1987). Despite the large number of studies on the nutritional deficiencies of low-income urban communities in developing countries, these analyses do not directly link the deficiencies to housing conditions or policy choices and tend to emphasize poverty as the underlying causal factor.

Mortality differentials within urban areas have also been linked with housing conditions. One recent study conducted in the shanty towns of Porto Alegre, Brazil (de Lima Guimaraes & Fischmann, 1985) showed that, while 20% of the city's infants lived in these settlements, 60% of the infants who died in 1980 were from shanty-town families, a majority of the deaths being attributable to intestinal diseases. The study drew on existing data, showing that intra-city differentials in mortality could be determined. The authors considered that a better targeting of health measures could be achieved with the aid of this kind of study. Although it suggested that poor environmental conditions were an underlying cause of the differentials in health status, the study did not propose any strategies to deal with these conditions, but concentrated instead on remedial action by the health services.

A study carried out in 1980–81 in Amman, Jordan (Tekce & Shorter, 1984) examined the socioeconomic and environmental factors associated with infant mortality in urban squatter settlements. The primary objectives of the study were to provide baseline data on the health conditions of the targeted populations for the planners of a five-settlement upgrading project, and to assess the potential of such a project to improve the health status of children. The authors concluded that the project would succeed in this aim because environmental conditions as well as household characteristics (maternal education in particular) were found to be significant determinants of child survival. However, the study assumed that the programme goals of tenure regularization and improvements in infrastructure and shelter would be achieved. The literature reviewed below suggests that unqualified success in a project is unlikely, and that a range of design and management factors can inhibit the improvement of health conditions.

The Agency for International Development has reviewed the epidemiological literature on housing and health and evaluated a variety of housing projects, including those conducted by its Office of Housing and Urban Development (USAID, 1981). Key components of the projects were examined, including water supply and storage, waste removal, provision of construction material, development of housing standards, urban gardening, and land-use planning. Municipal, national, and international policies related to the projects, such as financing, standard-setting, urban development initiatives, and employment generation, were not discussed. The report advocated better evaluation of the effects of housing programmes on health rather than new research on health and housing conditions. Methods for project evaluation and a framework for monitoring were proposed.

In 1987, WHO sponsored a consultation on the implications of housing for health (WHO, 1987a). The consultation analysed the links between housing and health, made recommendations for action to improve health conditions of housing, and approved a set of eleven "Health principles of housing", covering health needs, housing resource requirements, health policy, and community participation (WHO, 1989). The principles, which are presented in Table 5, are comprehensive and should prove useful in planning courses of action.

A recent review of community health and the urban poor (Harpham et al., 1988) examined the common health problems prevalent in poor urban communities, the delivery of primary health care and services, nutrition programmes, health education, sanitation, housing and integrated urban services. It included valuable case studies of government and community efforts to improve health conditions in various countries. In addition, the study reviewed a number of policy options for improving the health of low-income populations: targeting the poorest of the urban poor, introducing community diagnosis; ensuring better coordination between those serving the urban poor; and improving information on poor health conditions and their causes. To meet the needs of the urban poor more effectively, the authors advocated the scaling-up of pilot projects and the scaling-down of national health programmes to the local level.

Thus, the interrelationships between urban housing conditions and disease, infection, and behavioural problems are well documented, although a better understanding is still needed of the underlying causes of poor housing conditions. Pilot projects to improve conditions have been successful, but their duplication in an attempt to reach a greater proportion of the urban poor in developing countries has proved difficult. Problems in the implementation of government policy appear to be hindering the achievement of urban health objectives. Annis (1988) suggested that "today's urban technicians are generally to be found pondering a set of project options that—they believe—range from those that flatly make matters worse, to those that merely do not work very well, to those that work under restricted conditions but cannot be realistically financed or implemented on a wide scale".

Table 5. Health principles of housing

A. Principles related to health needs

1. Adequate housing provides protection against exposure to agents and vectors of communicable diseases, through
   - safe water supply,
   - sanitary excreta disposal,
   - disposal of solid wastes,
   - drainage of surface water,
   - personal and domestic hygiene,
   - safe food preparation, and
   - structural safeguards against disease transmission.

   1.1 An adequate supply of safe and potable water assists in preventing the spread of gastrointestinal diseases, supports domestic and personal hygiene, and provides an improved standard of living.

   1.2 Sanitary disposal of excreta reduces the faecal–oral transmission of disease and the breeding of insect vectors.

   1.3 Adequate and safe disposal of solid domestic wastes reduces health risks and helps to provide a more pleasant living environment; appropriate methods of storage and disposal discourage insect and rodent vectors of disease and protect people against poisonous substances and objects likely to cause accidental injury.

   1.4 Efficient drainage of surface waters helps to control communicable diseases, safety hazards, and damage to homes and property.

   1.5 Adequate housing includes facilities for personal and domestic hygiene, and people should be educated in hygienic practices.

   1.6 Healthy dwellings provide facilities for the safe preparation and storage of food, so that householders can employ sanitary food-handling practices.

   1.7 Adequate housing provides structural safeguards against the transmission of disease, including enough space to avoid overcrowding.

2. Adequate housing provides protection against injuries, poisonings, and thermal and other exposures that may contribute to chronic disease and malignancies; special attention should be paid to
   - structural features and furnishings,
   - indoor air pollution,
   - chemical safety, and
   - the use of the home as a workplace.

   2.1 The proper siting, structure, and furnishing of dwellings protect health, promote safety, and reduce hazards.

   2.2 Adequately designed, constructed, and ventilated dwellings, free of toxic and irritating substances, reduce the risks of chronic respiratory diseases and malignancies.

   2.3 Sensible precautions in the household reduce exposure to hazardous chemicals.

   2.4 Where a dwelling is also used as a workplace, those who live in it should be protected against hazards and contamination.

3. Adequate housing helps people's social and psychological development and reduces to a minimum the psychological and social stresses connected with the housing environment.
4. Suitable housing environments provide access to places of work, essential services, and amenities that promote good health.
5. Only if residents make proper use of housing can its health potential be realized to the full.

Table 5 (*continued*)

6. Housing should reduce to a minimum hazards to the health of groups at special risk from the conditions they live in, including
   - women and children,
   - those who live in substandard housing,
   - displaced and mobile populations, and
   - the aged, the chronically ill, and the disabled.

B. Principles related to health action

7. Health advocacy, carried out by health authorities and bodies in related fields, should be an integral part of public and private decisions about housing.
   7.1 Improvement of the health aspects of housing requires active leadership and informed advocacy by health authorities at all levels.
   7.2 Improved health in relation to housing can be served by mobilizing the energies and talents of all related agencies and groups.
   7.3 Health advocacy should work through a multiplicity of channels and media.
8. Economic and social policies that affect the state of housing should support the use of land and housing resources to maximize physical, mental, and social health.
9. Economic and social development, as it affects human shelter, should be based on appropriate processes of planning, the formulation and implementation of public policy, and the provision of services, with intersectoral collaboration in:
   - development planning and management,
   - urban and land-use planning,
   - housing legislation and standards and their enforcement,
   - the design and construction of housing,
   - the provision of community services, and
   - monitoring and surveillance of the situation.

   9.1. Incorporation of health and social criteria in the planning and management of economic development can prevent wasteful and dangerous housing being built.
   9.2. Taking social information and values into account in urban and land-use planning helps to ensure that housing will promote better health.
   9.3 Health requirements should be incorporated into legislation and standards that establish norms for the construction, maintenance, and use of dwellings and their surroundings. Such norms should be clear, consistent, and supportive of affordable, incrementally remedial housing provisions and made effective through adequate technical support services.
   9.4 Norms for housing design and construction technology should embody appropriate means of ensuring safety and promoting health.
   9.5 Sanitary and related health services should be organized in the community.
   9.6 Attainment of housing improvement goals requires active monitoring and surveillance.
10. Education—public and professional—should actively foster the provision and use of housing to promote health.
11. In dealing with the needs and problems of the human habitat, community involvement at all levels should support the processes of self-help, help between neighbours, and communal cooperative activities.

Source: WHO, 1989.

Housing policies for low-income populations

Urban housing policies receive considerable political attention at the national level, because housing is perhaps the most visible of all the problems associated with urbanization (Linn, 1984). With urban growth, the demand for urban labour does not expand as quickly as its supply, while the demand for urban housing and services expands more quickly than the supply (World Bank, 1983). Linn (1984) suggested that the poor suffer most directly from "maladjustments in the housing supply, in the form of loss of access to employment opportunities, poor health and nutrition, and general inconvenience".

In order to improve the supply of housing, governments intervene in a number of ways. Mayo et al. (1986) noted that they either apply direct measures, such as increasing the number of housing units, or take indirect action by providing funds, land, infrastructure, services, and/or materials, and by enforcing rent regulations, building codes, and building standards. Measures to improve the availability of housing and services for low-income populations have been adopted in the last two decades in most developing countries. The housing programmes reviewed below have all developed out of concern about the growth of inner-city slums, squatter settlements, and illegal subdivisions in cities throughout the developing world. Squatter settlements are characterized by illegal occupation of land, while the housing in illegal subdivisions is rented with the approval of the owners of the land, but not of the municipal authorities (Hardoy & Satterthwaite, 1986). The principal problems of people living in these areas are the high cost of housing, limited access to income, and the threat of forceable eviction (Hardoy & Satterthwaite, 1987).

Although some progress has been made in attending to the housing needs of low-income populations, a recent WHO survey of health authorities in developing countries revealed that under 50% of the countries surveyed had what was perceived as "a significant level of planning activity related to housing and socioeconomic development". In nearly all the countries surveyed, little baseline information was available on conditions, resources, and capacity to support planning efforts (WHO, 1987b).

Jorge E. Hardoy and David Satterthwaite have conducted the most extensive analyses of the links between health conditions and government action on urban issues. They have provided a useful classification of common government attitudes and action on urban housing problems, which consists of five stages ranging from disregard for the value of investment in providing low-income housing to recognition of the need for multisectoral approaches (such as health care provision and community self-help) to housing improvement. In most countries, the health authorities have not taken much part in urban planning. Little, if any, attention in housing planning is paid to the need for disease control and public health programmes (Hardoy, 1986). The World Bank (1983), in a review of urban programming and policies, noted the particular difficulty of handling "special components", such as health, nutrition, and community development, within housing and urban development schemes. The expertise required to manage and monitor such components is substantial and often beyond the resources of the administering authorities and assistance agencies. The competition between authorities and the "highly political character of existing social services in cities", suggested the World Bank report, also tended to lessen the opportunities for the successful inclusion of such components.

Problems in the implementation of housing policies are partly due to the way many administrative systems are organized. The implementation of these policies often "depends on a network of widely dispersed decision units whose responsibilities are also organizationally dispersed" (Grindle, 1980). Similarly, health services in urban areas are commonly provided by "a variety of ministries, social security organizations, municipal departments, quasi-governmental organizations, and private-sector institutions" (Rossi-Espagnet, 1987). The absence of coordinated administrative authority contributes to problems in the planning, monitoring, and evaluation of urban housing or health programmes (Hardoy & Satterthwaite, 1987; see also Jules-Rosette, 1988). Mayo et al. (1986) contended that governments often "misunderstand how the urban economy works and thus do not employ the right policies and programmes. This is especially true for housing."

The following review of the literature on housing clearance policies, the public provision of housing and services, sites-and-services projects, and programmes for upgrading slums and squatter settlements suggests that problems in the planning, implementation, and evaluation of major housing policies create significant health risks for the populations targeted.

Clearance of slums and squatter settlements

In the 1960s and early 1970s, the clearance of illegal squatter settlements was an accepted approach to urban housing problems. As Lacey & Owusu (1988) stated, in an analysis of housing policies in

Monrovia, Liberia, clearance and relocation strategies represent the "restrictive" approach to government involvement in housing problems. By restricting unauthorized building and service provision, planners thought that urban in-migration and overcrowding could be discouraged. Squatters removed from demolished settlements were resettled outside cities or on public lands within the city limits, moved to new government-constructed housing projects, or, more often than not, left to find shelter without public assistance.

While clearance removed some of the health hazards arising from conditions in squatter settlements, it created its own, perhaps more substantial, health problems. Community services developed by the residents, including the provision of water and even preventive health services, were curtailed, and substantial investments in shelter and community infrastructure destroyed. Clearance programmes also destroyed the complex community support systems often found in well established squatter settlements (Harpham et al., 1988; Linn, 1984).

Following clearance, former residents without access to public housing need to locate new low-cost sites and build there, which means having to scavenge or purchase costly materials. In the meantime, there is an increase in the serious risks to health associated with homelessness: little or no protection from the elements; lack of access to basic sanitation or water sources; inadequate nutrition due to the absence of cooking facilities and of money to buy prepared foods; and the spread of disease as a result of overcrowding in temporary accommodation (Harpham et al., 1988; Obudho & Mhlanga, 1988; Linn, 1984).

The failure of clearance policies to discourage urban migration or to encourage out-migration has led, in part, to their abandonment. More importantly, in many countries, the inevitable political repercussions of such policies were a powerful disincentive to this approach. The dispersion of large numbers of former squatters all over cities in search of new accommodation elicited protests from wealthier urban residents, while apparent disregard for the basic needs of squatters caused widespread criticism of government agencies and politicians. This criticism helped stimulate the creation of community organizations and nongovernmental agencies in numerous cities (Annis, 1988; Obudho & Mhlanga, 1988). Nevertheless, the clearance of settlements and the eviction of squatters have continued in some countries, creating new health risks and destroying valuable capital stock (Hardoy & Satterthwaite, 1986; Mayo et al., 1986). The spectre of eviction has proved a disincentive for the development of services and/or infrastructure to assist low-income settlement dwellers (Rossi-Espagnet, 1987).

Public provision of housing and infrastructure

When clearance schemes failed, many governments turned to more supportive housing policies (Lacey & Owusu, 1988). The most prominent alternative adopted in the 1970s was publicly constructed housing. Although the public construction of housing has helped, in some places, to meet the immediate needs of recent urban migrants and squatters, in most countries it has failed as a viable response to ever-increasing urban problems.

Public construction projects have generally failed to meet the long-term needs of the populations they serve, owing to population growth, excessive cost, and the inappropriate design of the housing and services provided (Obudho & Mhlanga, 1988). The cost is often high as a result of government inexperience, supply problems, and associated inefficiency. The high cost of building and the high standards applied have made many public housing programmes unaffordable for the populations targeted, so that projects have often benefited moderate-income rather than low-income groups (United Nations Centre for Human Settlements, 1988). For slum- or settlement-dwellers who cannot afford to move, little is available in the way of grants for improvements in existing housing, since housing funds are already fully allocated to building projects (Hardoy & Satterthwaite, 1986). Those who do move to public housing often find that the high cost forces them to adjust their spending. With resources depleted by the cost of housing, expenditure on items such as food may be threatened along with the nutritional status of households (Harpham et al., 1988). Public housing units are rarely in locations that are convenient to employment or to educational and health facilities (Hardoy, 1986); as a result, travel expenses go up and access to medical treatment is rendered difficult. The nature and severity of the effects of this situation on health are not well documented. At the moment, few housing projects require a baseline assessment of health conditions or of the concerns of people living in settlements or slums. There is thus little information on the possible contribution of these people to resolving health problems (Hardoy, 1986).

The role of the private sector in housing and the effects it has on health remain relatively unexplored. Linn (1984) considered that the private sector, with contributions from those to be served, tended to be more efficient and effective in providing housing than the public sector. While Mayo et al. (1986) agreed that the private sector could respond more quickly to housing demand, they argued that the public sector could make a greater effort to deal with inequalities in the housing market in order to achieve a fairer allocation of accommodation and services.

The provision of social services (including education, health, nutrition, and family planning services) is a politically sensitive issue, particularly in urban areas. Decisions on service areas, and the scope of the services to be provided, do not necessarily reflect the expressed or confirmed needs of low-income communities. Because health services require substantial initiation periods and capital investment, many projects aimed at providing health services may end up focusing on the building of clinics rather than on management, recurrent financing, or community outreach and prevention (Harpham et al., 1988; World Bank, 1983). In addition, low-income populations in urban areas are often faced with social and behavioural problems that require more complex social services than can be provided by primary health facilities or preventive health campaigns. To deal with alcohol abuse, drug use, mental illness, child abuse, and violence, which are rampant in many low-income urban communities, carefully developed counselling and rehabilitation programmes are required (Kayongo-Male, 1988). These needs are rarely met through the minimal medical services associated with public housing projects or welfare programmes.

The public provision of water, facilities for the disposal of sewage and solid wastes, and the related infrastructure has proved highly inadequate in most developing countries. In urban as well as rural areas, this situation is related to the lack of public capital financing for the installation of water and sanitation systems, and of recurrent financing for their maintenance as well as difficulties in measuring the costs and effectiveness of different approaches to the provision of water supplies (Harpham et al., 1988; Briscoe et al., 1986). While the question of the pricing of services is not explored here in depth, it has been suggested that failure to assess willingness to pay has led to underpricing and severely limited the resources available for extending services to low-income communities (Mayo et al., 1986). Linn (1984) noted that "inappropriate pricing policies have constrained public service investments and have encouraged overconsumption of services through subsidized prices for those households with access to services". The new service programmes developed in cooperation with private sector contractors in a numbers of developing countries may prove to be an important factor in extending services and reducing environmental health risks (Roth, 1987). Community involvement in the financing, construction, and maintenance of water and sanitation systems is another promising approach to the problem of ensuring greater sustainability of services (see Hasan, 1988). Hardoy (1986) contended that education in hygiene and disease control should go hand-in-hand with water and sanitation programmes, if improvements in health status are to be achieved.

The positive effects of water supply and sanitation schemes on the health of the populations covered have not yet been adequately documented, although some studies on the subject exist (Wang et al., 1989; Planas, 1988; Briscoe, 1987; Briscoe et al., 1986; Esrey et al., 1985). Evidence of an independent cause-and-effect mechanism is still slim. The methodological difficulties involved in evaluating the effects of water supply, sanitation, and education in hygiene have been carefully analysed and discussed by Briscoe et al. (1986). Their report suggested improvements in the design of health impact evaluations, including the increased use of the case–control method and rapid assessments to provide information for policy decisions (see Briscoe et al., 1988, for an evaluation of the case–control method in Africa and Asia). The development of water supply policies that can substantially improve health conditions will depend on better research to determine key factors that could make such policies cost-effective and sustainable.

Sites-and-services programmes

Given the frequent failure of public housing programmes, many governments have shifted their attention to the provision of plots with basic services foı former squatters or slum residents and new migrants, who are then given assistance in building their own homes. The increasingly favoured sites-and-services approach has been adopted by many developing countries over the last two decades with the assistance of international agencies such as the World Bank. The major objectives of this approach, as well as the upgrading approach described below, are to make housing more affordable, enable more of the project costs to be recovered, and promote community self-help (Mayo et al., 1986). Many sites-and-services programmes have, at least in the short run, reduced overcrowding, improved access to certain services, and encouraged infrastructural development. Through these approaches, some of the most significant environmental health risks for the targeted groups may be reduced (Harpham et al., 1988; Obudho & Mhlanga, 1988; Lacey & Owusu, 1988; WHO, 1987a).

Planning and management problems have, however, restricted the participation of the targeted groups and prevented the programmes from meeting long-term needs, such as the alleviation of environmental health hazards. The land provided for sites-and-services projects has often been inadequate or inconveniently located, making it difficult to extend services, such as water supply and sewerage, and increasing transport costs for residents (Hardoy, 1986). The projects have failed to recover costs to the extent anticipated, thus reducing resources for their expansion (United Nations Centre for Human Settlements, 1988; Payne, 1984; Burgess, 1985). Building credits and assistance are initially available, but credit resources tend to run short of demand. Building and service costs may exceed those predicted and are often beyond the means of the low-income groups targeted (Mayo et al., 1986; Hardoy, 1986). One result has been the leakage of project benefits to moderate-income groups who can cover costs. Nientied & van der Linden (1988) argue that in many countries there is strong evidence that important political, administrative, and economic interests favour this maldistribution of benefits and wish to restrict the expansion of programmes serving the very poor.

Even when the objective is to improve the range and quality of housing for low-income communities, problems of project design have created additional costs for the intended beneficiaries. Mayo et al. (1986) contended that planners of sites-and-services programmes, as well as international funding agencies, had contributed to the failure of many such programmes, by making incorrect assumptions regarding the percentage of the budget in low-income households available to meet housing expenses. Their research concluded that the commonly accepted figure of 20–25% underestimated actual spending behaviour. Many intended participants in housing programmes, therefore, require government subsidies in order to build and maintain their homes. These unexpected financial outlays are likely to restrict the replication of such programmes.

To increase access to programmes and make them more sustainable, Mayo et al. (1986) advocated improvements in mechanisms for financing housing, including loan programmes with more realistic interest rates. Innovative sources of credit, such as community contributions and revolving funds, also need to be identified and made available (Obudho & Mhlanga, 1988; Harpham et al., 1988; Mayo et al., 1986). Even when it has been made possible for them to build, participants in the project may choose to sell their sites to better-off buyers for immediate financial gain. The sellers may then seek out alternative low-cost housing in other squatter settlements, foregoing opportunities for improved services and shelter (Amis, 1984; Gilbert & Gugler, 1981). More analysis is required to assess whether their gains lead to short-term improvements in household resources and food consumption, and whether the commercialization of the sites has long-term positive or negative effects on health.

Programme implementation, in many cases, may create additional obstacles for the participants. Information and management problems are particularly severe in many sites-and-services projects. Procedures for obtaining loans may be unduly complicated, and information on financing, credit, low-cost building materials, and technical assistance may not be readily available (see Kayongo-Male, 1988; Jules-Rosette, 1988). Households headed by women experience particular difficulty in meeting the requirements for participation, since they may not be able to demonstrate that they have stable incomes (Hardoy & Satterthwaite, 1986). Moser & Peake (1987) edited a thorough review of the problems confronting women in low-income housing programmes in a variety of developing countries. It often proves impossible to keep to the building timetables established by programme developers and lenders (Hardoy & Satterthwaite, 1986). Delays in implementation tend to plague projects, sometimes leading to the closure of services in squatter settlements long before new housing units are ready for occupancy and before new services can be provided (Muller, 1988). In the interim periods, residents may again be confronted with environmental health problems that had been successfully dealt with through community action before the projects began. An analysis of the nature and scope of the hazards and ill-health associated with such time-lags, and suggestions on how to avoid them, would be useful.

Even when new programmes do meet the immediate needs of the targeted groups with regard to shelter, infrastructure, and services, they often fail to allow for the additional population attracted to the community by the programmes. Renewed overcrowding can result, and health conditions can deteriorate (Lacey & Owusu, 1988). In an evaluation of a sites-and-services project in Lusaka, Zambia, supported by the World Bank, the authors found little evidence to suggest that in-migration had increased as a result of the project. However, they noted that plots in former squatter settlements abandoned by the participants in the project were quickly occupied by new migrants (Bamberger et al., 1982). Thus, urban planning for current and future community needs requires more than a project-by-project approach.

Certain recent initiatives may help to alleviate mismanagement and confusion in these projects, notably the preparation of an administrative and operational guide for sites-and-services in Botswana, in cooperation with the World Bank (Campbell, 1985). Given the peculiarities of national policies and local conditions, similar guides will undoubtedly need to be developed for specific country programmes. The Botswana guide and other evaluations of sites-

and-services projects do not deal explicitly with measures to achieve better results from the health standpoint or to facilitate the provision of health services in connection with the projects. Because of failure to collect baseline data, evaluations have been unable to demonstrate changes in health conditions directly linked to sites-and-services projects (Bamberger et al., 1982). While improved management is likely to make them more successful, inadequacy of resources and lack of cooperation between the government and the community will continue to hinder the ability of such projects to meet the long-term housing and service needs of poor urban communities.

Upgrading of slums and squatter settlements

It is estimated that 86% of housing stock is produced by the informal sector in the Philippines, 82% in Brazil, and 77% in Venezuela (United Nations Centre for Human Settlements, 1988). Housing in illegal subdivisions, squatter settlements, and slums has developed and expanded through individual initiatives as well as through building groups, cooperatives, and community associations (United States Centre for Human Settlements, 1988). By the mid-1970s it was evident that, by supporting such self-help initiatives, governments could forge ahead with the provision of housing and services, while saving on costs (Hardoy, 1986). Programmes for the upgrading of slums and squatter settlements are based on this approach, which is capable of reaching a larger proportion of the urban poor than other housing strategies and has led to substantial improvements in health conditions (World Health Organization, 1987b). International assistance agencies have continued to favour the self-help approach and have contributed substantially to upgrading programmes.

Upgrading programmes aim to build on the work and investments of existing slum and squatter communities, whether legal or illegal, by adding much needed materials and services. As with sites-and-services programmes, they help to increase access to building credit and the provision of basic infrastructure and services, often with the cooperation and contributions of members of the community. Other upgrading measures include better access for vehicles, land or structural stabilization, and technical assistance (WHO, 1987b). Most upgrading programmes are designed to carry out measures that are requested by residents and within their means.

One of the most important features of upgrading programmes is the improved security of tenure achieved through the legalization of existing settlements or subdivisions and the apportionment of land titles (Harpham et al., 1988; WHO, 1987b; Obudho & Mhlanga,

1988). Such measures often require the modification of existing laws, policies, and institutional practices (Hardoy & Satterthwaite, 1986). However, the legalization of property can have unintended consequences. Low-income squatters and renters may be displaced by moderate-income groups attracted by the newly commercialized properties (Satterthwaite, 1986). In addition, legalization tends to exclude some of the settlement-dwellers and to restrict the future growth of settlements, so that some low-income families are displaced and the entrance of others is restricted (Nientied & van der Linden, 1988; Amis, 1984; Gilbert & Gugler, 1981).

The literature suggests that upgrading programmes have been ineffective in providing direct measures to reduce ill-health. Hardoy (1986) stated that "rarely has there been a careful assessment of how an upgrading programme can best improve health and control disease", in part because housing planners and builders are lacking in health awareness. The extension of services is often restricted by the location of settlements and other problems, and expected health improvements are limited as a result. Physical obstacles, such as poor subsoil quality, lack of roads, or sheer distance from mains pipes and energy sources may prevent the provision of water, sewerage systems, or electricity. The steady supply of water or electricity may also be obstructed by the poor quality of extension projects, lack of maintenance, and interference with supply lines (Hardoy, 1986). The displacement and disruption resulting from the installation of services may create new environmental health risks in the short run, and the water supply or sewerage infrastructure can reduce space for shelter in the long run (S. Angel, personal communication, 1989).

The delivery of health care may also continue to be limited after upgrading begins. Health workers may not have easy access to settlements, and residents may continue to lack access to services in central districts unless upgrading is accompanied by the provision of new public transport services, which is rare. Thus, improvements in infrastructure and services have often been insufficient to reduce environmental hazards or improve health conditions significantly (Obudho & Mhlanga, 1988). There are examples of upgrading programmes that have included successful health components, such as primary care, maternal and child services, nutrition, family planning, and training of community health workers, in Addis Ababa, Hyderabad, Kuala Lumpur, Lima, Lusaka, Rio de Janeiro, and other cities (see case-studies presented in Harpham et al., 1988; Rossi-Espagnet, 1987). Gardening projects to increase food resources have also proved successful in some urban areas (Sanyal, 1985; USAID, 1981). However, most initiatives have succeeded only at the level of individual projects so far, and have not been replicated across cities or regions.

The composition and scale of squatter settlements have changed over recent decades in most developing countries. These communities have become complex mixtures of "residents, owners, resident landlords, absentee landlords, government-owned plots, municipal council plots" (Kayongo-Male, 1988). As a result, upgrading programmes have become difficult to manage and difficult to target at those residents most in need. More extensive services and more elaborate planning are required. If health conditions in the settlements are to continue to improve, increased long-term financial support for upgrading projects is needed, together with the provision of low-cost materials and the training of community residents to maintain systems and provide basic services.

In both upgrading projects and sites-and-services projects, the cross-subsidization of plot charges may help increase funding for infrastructure and utilities: people identified as having a greater ability to pay are charged higher plot prices, and the excess funds used to subsidize the needs of poorer residents (Linn, 1984). This may compensate somewhat for the leakage of benefits associated with both upgrading and sites-and-services projects. Given the difficulties of targeting, cross-subsidization schemes may help poorer residents to benefit from the inevitable mixture of populations. Although there is no record of it as yet, these schemes may contribute to efforts to help remove health hazards through the community financing of public services, such as water supply, sanitation, and road-building.

The success of programme implementation often depends on the power and force of community demands (Annis, 1988; Obudho & Mhlanga, 1988). Recent analyses of urban policy-making in developing countries suggest that the urban poor are increasingly prepared to organize themselves, assess their own needs, and voice their concerns in the political sphere (Annis, 1988; Rossi-Espagnet, 1987; Peattie & Aldrete-Haas, 1981). In Mexico, nongovernmental agencies working with community organizers and tenants' groups have proved highly successful in directing government resources to housing and service programmes and to community self-help efforts (Annis, 1988). However, in some communities, particularly in Africa, political organization may not be easily achieved, overt confrontation may be frowned upon, and felt needs may rarely be openly expressed (see Kayongo-Male, 1988).

Slum-upgrading programmes have become noted for their ability to preserve community dynamics that have developed over the years and for their active encouragement and use of community participation (Linn, 1984). Upgrading policies and programmes that assume community commitment and interest, however, may fail to achieve their welfare objectives. Researchers in Ghana found that some squatter settlements had deteriorated, owing to the instability of their populations and the absence of community action. Upgrading programmes were not accepted in these settlements, and alternative programmes in new locations were necessary to meet the needs of the residents (Tipple, 1988). The World Health Organization (WHO, 1987b) has produced a guide on the improvement of environmental health conditions in low-income urban settlements, using a "community-based approach to identifying needs and priorities". This guide describes methods for community-based surveys and makes recommendations for community participation and action, which are viewed as essential to the proper development of upgrading programmes. An evaluation of the effectiveness of community-based assessment and planning measures in programme development would be useful.

Standard-setting and regulatory measures

In recent years, both standard-setting and regulatory measures to control housing conditions in urban areas have come in for a great deal of criticism. Inappropriate standards, codes, and zoning regulations have hampered both sites-and-services and upgrading programmes. Standards and regulations from industrial countries have often been adopted and employed to protect the health and safety of wealthy urban communities (Rossi-Espagnet, 1987). Their enforcement has done a great deal to restrict efforts to improve the health of low-income populations. Instead of expanding the availability of affordable and safe housing, standards and regulations can reduce the amount of housing stock accessible to low-income groups and increase building costs (Mayo et al., 1986). They can also create a fresh risk of eviction for people living in substandard housing. In sites-and-services and upgrading projects, the potential beneficiaries often need government subsidies to purchase the high-cost building materials needed in order to comply with standards. Thus, standards may increase government spending and reduce the sustainability of housing programmes or reduce the pool of beneficiaries (Mayo et al., 1986). Another matter requiring attention is the part played by bribery and corruption in establishing standards and relaxing enforcement, and the effect on household resources of the under-the-table deals involved.

The enforcement of strict standards has also inhibited improvements in sanitation. In many countries, the introduction of modern sewerage systems is not feasible owing to lack of resources, topographic obstacles, and the risk of community disruption in the construction phase. While pit or pour-flush latrines have been widely advocated as viable alternatives to modern piped sanitation, they have not proved politically or culturally acceptable in many countries. The United Nations Centre for Human Settlements (1988) suggested that educational campaigns were needed to facilitate the acceptance of new basic technologies.

Zoning and population density limits are often formulated to rule out the development of squatter communities in inner-city districts and in areas considered inappropriate for the extension of public services. However, zoning measures may have the effect of eliminating the only land and housing opportunities open to new migrants, since most other land is acquired by major commercial interests or controlled by private real estate developers. When settlements do develop, the zoning restrictions can ensure that the legal extension of infrastructure and services will be prohibited (Obudho & Mhlanga, 1988). In some countries, such as Brazil and Sri Lanka, progress has been made in modifying standards, zoning, and choice of technology in projects for the provision of housing and services (Rossi-Espagnet, 1987). Nevertheless, these countries appear to be the exception rather than the rule.

The World Health Organization, the World Bank, and housing advocates in developing countries have called for the development of flexible standards that will fit the needs both of builders and of future tenants, without sacrificing either quality or safety (WHO, 1987a; Hardoy & Satterthwaite, 1987; Mayo et al., 1986). These would allow for community decision-making and improve access to low-cost, locally available materials and sites. The resulting housing conditions would reduce the health risks associated with homelessness and unserviced makeshift housing, without leading to economic hardship. The lack of precise data on housing conditions, enforcement measures, and manpower will continue to be a major obstacle to the development and application of appropriate regulations and controls.

Mayo et al. (1986) suggested that attention should be centred on housing input markets (e.g., land and building materials) rather than the production process (e.g., housing standards). Most analysts of urban health conditions agree. Improvements in security of tenure, building credits and materials, and infrastructure are considered to be more effective in reducing health risks than overambitious quality standards. At the same time, more epidemiological research is required to determine the building materials and designs that will reduce household health hazards most effectively and efficiently.

Conclusion

Even with strong evidence of the links between housing and health and a commitment to serving low-income populations, governments have encountered a great many difficulties in their efforts to improve environmental health. Although notable progress has been made in extending programmes to help poor urban communities, housing policies have often had unintended negative effects on the living conditions, health status, and economic security of the poor. The cost to health of temporary or permanent displacement, the straining of household budgets, and the leakage of project resources may be substantial. Owing to the lack of data on the costs and benefits of specific sites-and-services projects and slum-upgrading efforts in terms of health, it is impossible to determine the extent to which they have improved health conditions in poor urban communities or to estimate the scope of the new health risks they have created.

Programme difficulties are due, in the first place, to inadequacies of information, needs assessment, planning, and evaluation. The absence of baseline data on health conditions hinders the development of appropriate health and environmental programmes as well as the evaluation of the results. Because needs have been inadequately assessed, planners have had little sense of actual housing demand, community resources, or willingness to pay for housing and infrastructure. Prospective case–control or cross-sectional studies would be helpful in identifying and quantifying the health effects, both positive and negative, of the various programme activities. In addition, studies to assess their social impact would help uncover problems of household employment, spending, and community disruption, that might create health risks in the future.

Urban housing and health conditions may not be significantly improved through policies that provide only minimal support for the purchase of land and the building of homes, without concomitant improvements in the provision of services. Sites-and-services projects and upgrading programmes may not go far enough in providing low-income urban communities with the foundations for sustainable basic services, including water, sanitation, solid-waste disposal, education, and public health services. A lack of coordination between housing and health authorities and a scarcity of resources for broad-based primary care, disease control, and community outreach restrict improvements in health conditions still further.

Housing programmes have also proved incapable of preventing the leakage of benefits from the poorest urban residents to groups with greater disposable incomes. Better targeting will need to be accompanied by efforts to reduce building and maintenance costs, and by more efficient and effective provision of public services. Where restrictive targeting is not feasible, cross-subsidization involving the use of rents from higher-income households to help cover housing and service costs for lower-income households may be a promising option. An equitable means of charging users for services may also be required. The involvement of service contractors and communities themselves in the provision and maintenance of services may help reduce the inefficiencies associated with government efforts in this area.

Both health analysts and housing analysts strongly support housing policies that apply appropriate housing standards, provide secure land tenure, and promote self-help housing and infrastructure development. Ways of enhancing the feasibility, and improving the implementation, of such policies are now required. Poor implementation has frequently impeded projects to improve health conditions. Better programme management, financing, and institutional coordination are required to help mitigate unintended effects on health and to expand direct health promotion efforts. An infusion of management expertise, planning, and technical assistance appears to be essential, as does the improved training of programme managers in health impact assessment. Explicit policies aimed at improving management skills in the public services may be as important as basic programme planning and financing.

Even if problems of project planning and implementation are surmounted, sites-and-services projects and upgrading programmes will need to be expanded, in order to meet the long-term housing and health needs of poor urban populations at their current rate of growth in many developing countries. The health concerns of low-income populations need to be addressed directly, and community participation must be ensured.

References

Amis, P. (1984) Squatters or tenants—the commercialization of unauthorized housing in Nairobi. *World development*, 12(1): 87–96.

Annis, S. (1988) What is not the same about the urban poor: the case of Mexico City. In: *Strengthening the poor: what have we learned.* New Brunswick, Transaction Books (for the Overseas Development Council).

Bamberger, M. et al. (1982) *Evaluation of sites and services projects: the experience from Lusaka, Zambia*. Washington, DC, World Bank (Staff Working Paper No. 548).

Basta, S. S. (1982) Health programmes directed to urban squatter populations. In: Taylor, J. L. & Williams, D. G., ed. *Urban planning practice in developing countries*, Oxford, Pergamon Press.

Basta, S. S. (1977) Nutrition and health in low income urban areas of the Third World. *Ecology of food and nutrition*, **6**: 113–124.

Briscoe, J. (1987) A role for water supply and sanitation in the child survival revolution. *Bulletin of the Pan American Health Organization*, **2**(2): 93–105.

Briscoe, J. et al. (1986) *Evaluating health impact: water supply, sanitation, and hygiene education*. Ottawa, International Development Research Centre.

Briscoe, J. et al. (1988) Case-control studies of the effect of environmental sanitation on diarrhoea morbidity: methodological implications of field studies in Africa and Asia. *International journal of epidemiology*, **17**(2): 441–447.

Burgess, R. (1985) The limits to state self-help housing programmes. *Development and change*, **16**: 271–312.

Campbell, J. R. , ed. (1985) *Administrative and operational procedures for programs for sites and services and area upgrading*. Washington, DC, World Bank.

Data Banik, N. D. (1977) Some observations on feeding programmes, nutrition and growth of preschool children in an urban community. *Indian journal of pediatrics*, **44**(353): 139–149.

Data Banik, N. D. (1979) Feeding habits and weaning practices in infants and preschool children in slum areas in New Delhi. *Archives of child health*, **21**(3): 51–57.

de la Luz Alvarez, M. et al. (1979) Caracteristicas de familias urbanas con lactantes, desnutridos. *Achivos latinoamericanos de nutrición*, **29**(2): 220–232.

de Lima Guimaraes, J. J. & Fischmann, A. (1985) Inequalities in 1980: infant mortality among shantytown residents and nonshantytown residents in the municipality of Porto Alegre, Rio Grande Do Sul, Brazil. *Bulletin of the Pan American Health Organization*, **19**(3): 235–251.

Esrey, S. A. et al. (1985) Interventions for the control of diarrhoeal diseases among young children: improving water supplies and excreta disposal facilities. *Bulletin of the World Health Organization*, **63**(4): 757–772.

Gilbert, A. & Gugler, J. (1981) *Cities, poverty, and development: urbanization in the Third World*. New York, Oxford University Press.

Grindle, M. (1980) Policy content and context in implementation. In: Grindle, M. , ed. *Politics and policy implementation in the Third World*. Princeton, Princeton University Press.

Hardoy, J. E. (1986) Habitat and health: an exploration of their interrelationship. In: Tulchin, J. S. , ed. *Habitat, health, and development*. Boulder, CO, Lynne Reiner Publishers.

Hardoy, J. E. & Satterthwaite, D. (1986) Shelter, infrastructure and services in Third World cities. *Habitat international*, **10**(3): 245–284.

Hardoy, J. E. & Satterthwaite, D. (1987) Housing and health: do architects and planners have a role? *Cities*, **4**(3): 221–235.

Harpham, T. et al. (1988) *In the shadow of the city: community health and the urban poor*. Oxford, Oxford University Press.

Hasan, A. (1988) Low-cost sanitation for a squatter community. *World health forum*, **9**: 361–364.

Hussain, A. M. & Lunven, P. (1987) Urbanization and hunger in the cities. *Food and nutrition bulletin*, **9**(4): 50–61.

Jensen, L. (1988) Developing countries begin grappling with urban woes. *World development*, **1**(4): 4–8.

Jules-Rosette, B. (1988) A Zambian squatter complex: cultural variables in urban relocation. In: Obudho, R. A. & Mhlanga, C. C., ed. *Slum and squatter settlements in sub-Saharan Africa: toward a planning strategy*. New York, Praeger.

Kayongo-Male, D. (1988) Slum and squatter settlements in Kenya: housing problems and planning possibilities. In: Obudho, R. A. & Mhlanga, C. C., ed. *Slum and squatter settlements in sub-Saharan Africa: toward a planning strategy*. New York, Praeger.

Kerejan, H. & N'da, K. (1981) Approches des problèmes alimentaires et nutritionnels d'une mégalopole africaine. *Médecine d' Afrique noire*, **28**(7): 479–482.

Lacey, L. & Owusu, S. E. (1988) Squatter settlements in Monrovia, Liberia: the evolution of housing policies. In: Obudho, R. A. & Mhlanga, C. C., ed. *Slum and squatter settlements in sub-Saharan Africa: toward a planning strategy*. New York, Praeger.

Linn, J. F. (1984) *Cities in the developing world: policies for their equitable and efficient growth*. New York, Oxford University Press (for the World Bank).

Martin, A. E. et al. (1976) *Housing, the housing environment, and health*. Geneva, World Health Organization (Offset Publication No. 27).

Mayo, S. K. et al. (1986) Shelter strategies for the urban poor in developing countries. *Research observer*, **1**(2): 183–203.

Michelina, A. (1988) *Social policies and health*. Report of the ILPES-PAHO-CORDIPLAN project, submitted to the Pan American Health Organization.

Moser, C. O. N. & Peake, L., ed. (1987) *Women, human settlements and housing*. London, Tavistock Publications.

Muller, M. S. (1988) The improvement of Chawama, a squatter settlement in Lusaka, Zambia. In: Obudho, R. A. & Mhlanga, C. C., ed. *Slum and squatter settlements in sub-Saharan Africa: toward a planning strategy*. New York, Praeger.

Nientied, P. & van der Linden, J. (1988) The "new" policy approach to housing: a review of the literature. *Public administration and development*, **8**: 233–240.

Obudho, R. A. & Mhlanga, C. C. (1988) Planning strategies for slum and squatter settlements in sub-Saharan Africa. In: Obudho, R. A. &

Mhlanga, C. C., ed. *Slum and squatter settlements in sub-Saharan Africa: toward a planning strategy*. New York, Praeger.

Payne, G., ed. (1984) *Low-income housing in the developing world: the role of sites and services and settlement upgrading*. Chichester, John Wiley.

Peattie, L. & Aldrete-Haas, J. A. (1981) "Marginal" settlements in developing countries. *Annual review of sociology*, 7: 157–175.

Planas, A. (1988) Implementation of the drinking water supply and sanitation decade in Latin America and the Caribbean. *Natural resources forum*, **12**(3): 255–266.

Popkin, B. M. & Bisgrove, E. Z. (1988) Urbanization and nutrition in low-income countries. *Food and nutrition bulletin*, **10**(1): 3–23.

Rossi-Espagnet, A. (1987) Health services and environmental factors in urban slums and shanty towns of the developing world. *Food and nutrition bulletin*, **9**(4): 4–20.

Roth, G. (1987) *The private provision of public services in developing countries*. New York, Oxford University Press (for the World Bank).

Sanyal, B. (1985) Urban agriculture: who cultivates and why? A case-study of Lusaka, Zambia. *Food and nutrition bulletin*, 7(3): 15–24.

Satterthwaite, D. (1984) Preventive planning: what are we planning to prevent?. In: Tulchin, J. S., ed. *Habitat, health, and development*. Boulder, CO, Lynne Reiner Publishers.

Sigulem, D. M. & Tudisco, E. S. (1980) Aleitamento natural en diferentes classes de renda no municipio de São Paulo. *Archivos latinoamericanos de nutrición*, **30**(3): 400–416.

Stephens, B. et al. (1985). Health and low-cost housing. *World health forum*, **6**: 59–62.

Tekce, B. & Shorter, F. C. (1984) Determinants of child mortality: a study of squatter settlements in Jordan. In: *Child survival: strategies for research*. Supplement to: *Population and development review*, **10**: 257–280.

Tipple, A. G. (1988) Upgrading and culture in Kumasi: problems and possibilities. In: Obudho, R. A. & Mhlanga, C. C., ed. *Slum and squatter settlements in sub-Saharan Africa: toward a planning strategy*. New York, Praeger.

United Nations Centre for Human Settlements (Habitat) (1988) *Health implications of public policies for the housing sector*. Paper presented at the Healthy Public Policy Conference, sponsored by the Australian Commonwealth Department of Health and the World Health Organization, Adelaide, Australia.

USAID (1981). Office of Housing and Urban Development. *Housing and health: an analysis for use in the planning, design and evaluation of low-income housing programs*. Washington, DC, US Agency for International Development.

Viteri, F. E. (1987) Nutrition-related health consequences of urbanization. *Food and nutrition bulletin*, **8**(4): 33–49.

Wang, Z. S. et al. (1989) Reduction of enteric infectious disease in rural China by providing deep-well tap water. *Bulletin of the World Health Organization*, **67**: 171–180.

WHO (1987a) *Housing —the implications for health. Report of a WHO consultation.* Unpublished WHO document WHO/EHE/RUD/87. 2.
WHO (1987b) *Improving environmental health conditions in low-income settlements: a community-based approach to identifying needs and priorities.* Geneva, World Health Organization (Offset Publication No. 100).
WHO (1989) *Health principles of housing.* Geneva, World Health Organization.
World Bank (1983) *Learning by doing: World Bank lending for urban development, 1972–1982.* Washington, DC.

CHAPTER 7

Conclusions

The literature on the effects of development policies on health covers many disciplinary fields, substantive questions, and government authorities. This review has identified some key documents for each sector of development. At the same time, it has demonstrated that a sizable, but rather unsatisfactory, literature exists at the intersection of development policies and health conditions. For each sector, it has discussed gaps in knowledge about the effects of policy on health, and the measures available to mitigate negative effects and improve health conditions. The relevant findings in both areas are summarized in the conclusions at the end of each chapter.

Overall, this review has led to three major conclusions:

(1) Analyses and evaluations of development policies tend not to examine the implications for health.

(2) Research on health problems in developing countries tends to ignore the role of development policies as an underlying cause of ill-health.

(3) Even when knowledge and good documentation exist on the effects of development policies on health, numerous obstacles (technical, institutional, and political) can still hinder the effective implementation of policy changes to improve health.

These themes are discussed below, with illustrations from each sector of development.

Failure to analyse health consequences

As regards macroeconomic policies, some efforts have been made to consider their effects on health, mainly as they result from reductions in public expenditure on social services. The effects of cutbacks in public spending, which are associated with adjustment policies, are described in terms of greater morbidity and, sometimes, higher infant mortality, of acute shortages of pharmaceutical and medical supplies, and of reduced health capital stock (for example, clinics and equipment). Studies of other macroeconomic policies tend to include assessments of their effects on the nutritional status of households but rarely deal with the resulting changes in health conditions. More work needs to be done in this area. The policies in question include food pricing, food subsidies and programmes, and the promotion of export crop production. The literature does not provide a clear explanation for the emphasis on nutritional rather than health indicators, but this may be partly due to methodological constraints. Difficulties exist, especially in measuring the health effects of nutritional decline and in quantifying changes in health conditions attributable solely to macroeconomic policies. In the past decade, greater attention has been paid to analysing increases in morbidity and mortality associated with adjustment policies, and some analysts believe the available evidence is sufficiently strong to warrant changes in macroeconomic policies.

Analyses of agricultural policy have similarly tended not to look at the effects on health, except in the area of water resource development, where an association with vector-borne diseases is now recognized, after over two decades of prompting by a number of agencies. Although irrigation development schemes nowadays often require rapid assessments of risks to health, few projects actually carry out careful pre- and post-implementation surveys of the incidence of specific vector-borne and other water-related diseases (such as malaria, schistosomiasis, and Japanese encephalitis). Government subsidies for pesticides, which are intended to increase agricultural productivity, have not been examined from the health standpoint, although various harmful consequences of increased pesticide use are well documented: accidental poisoning of the producers who apply the chemicals; accidental poisoning of consumers who may ingest the chemicals; increased resistance of disease vectors to pesticides; and over-reliance on chemical pest-control strategies when other measures (such as integrated pest management) might be applied more safely and at lower cost. Further evaluation is required to assess which approaches are most suitable to local conditions. Policies intended to change conditions of land tenure have rarely taken into account the potential effects on health —as, for example, in the case of new migrants attracted to tropical regions where malaria is endemic. Finally, agricultural researchers have only begun to consider how their priorities and decisions about the development of new agricultural technologies could affect the health and nutrition of farming families and consumers.

The literature on industrial policies has emphasized the consequences of government intervention for economic growth and general social welfare, with relatively little attention to the consequences for health. Analyses of the harmful effects on the environment of industrial policies that encourage certain patterns of specialization, ownership, and siting, have generally failed to consider the short-term and long-term implications for health. In part, this shortcoming may be due to the lack of evidence of clear cause-and-effect relationships as well as the tendency to neglect the health angle in the development of industrial policies. Policies to encourage small-scale enterprises and activities in the informal sector have similarly disregarded the potential adverse effects on the health of the low-income workers employed there and the adjacent communities. Although increasing attention is being paid to health conditions inside factories, the consequences for communities in areas of industrial development remain a low priority in the design and analysis of industrial policies. Growing awareness of the scope and effects of air and water pollution, and of hazardous waste, has greatly increased the role of policy-makers in pollution control in developing countries. Nevertheless, an effort must be made to assess the implications of new industrial regulations as regards the improvement or exacerbation of health conditions for those most heavily exposed to sources of pollution.

Analyses of energy policies in developing countries have not paid sufficient attention to the effects of energy extraction, consumption, and pricing on health. Deforestation appears to be threatening the nutritional and health status of poor households as a result of the increase in the time spent by women in collecting firewood and the reduction in energy resources for food preparation. But policies to increase reserves of wood fuel have rarely touched the households that suffer most from fuel poverty. Concern for fuel scarcity has led to efforts to make the domestic use of fuel more efficient, but it is only recently that attention has been paid to the improvements in cooking-stoves and housing needed to reduce the health risks presented by the combustion of biofuels. Fuel-pricing strategies and subsidies have not taken effects on health into consideration or intentionally promoted safe fuels, and pricing decisions may favour urban populations over their rural counterparts. Hydropower development is high on the agenda of most planners in the energy sector, with continued emphasis on large dams. Unfortunately, the health risks and costs associated with the proliferation of this type of undertaking still do not figure prominently in feasibility studies, the project approval process or project implementation.

As regards housing policies, a considerable literature exists on the health effects of government intervention. Analyses of urban housing policies, however, rarely pay adequate attention to the baseline health conditions of the low-income populations targeted. And evaluations of housing programmes rarely assess changes in the health conditions of the populations served. This situation may be due to the numerous complicating factors that affect the relationship between housing and health, including income, employment, and educational level as well as the social dynamics and behavioural patterns of urban life (i.e., such factors as sexually transmitted diseases, substance abuse, child abuse, stress-related illness, and inadequate nutritional intake due to preferential expenditure on alcohol or luxury items). Nevertheless, a number of recent reports have provided specific recommendations on ways of improving assessments of effects on health and incorporating health considerations in urban housing policies.

Need for more analyses of development policy

For the past several decades, studies of health and development have emphasized poverty as a cause of disease and death. At the same time, greater equity and less poverty have been prominent goals of development policy, even if more in rhetoric than in achievement. Until the 1980s, analyses of health problems in developing countries did not generally consider macroeconomic policy as an important factor. In the past decade, however, the debt crisis of developing countries and the subsequent adjustment programmes have led to a change of perspective. UNICEF in particular, but other organizations and individuals as well, undertook analyses of adjustment policies and strongly criticized their negative impact on the health and nutrition of poor populations in developing countries. On the basis of social impact research, the following specific changes in macroeconomic policy were proposed with a view to alleviating the negative consequences: better targeting of food subsidies; restructuring of public expenditure to protect key programmes in the health sector; and an increase in employment programmes for the poor. Some countries and donors have begun to support such measures, but many difficulties remain. The problem of implementing restructuring and adjustment policies without producing increased hardship for the poor is still far from solved. On the whole, health research has remained ineffective in analysing macroeconomic policies and in influencing the choice of specific macroeconomic policies.

As regards the agricultural sector, health analysts have a long history of examining the consequences of irrigation projects in terms of disease. Yet, better analysis could be carried out of the objectives of, and incentives for, specific types of irrigation policy, and the modifications needed to reduce their adverse effects on health. In the case of pesticides, epidemiological analysis has been primarily concerned with documenting the existence and immediate causes of acute poisoning, and has not directly connected these with government policies promoting pesticide production and subsidization. While alternatives to the use of pesticides have been identified, and their benefits weighed, little attention has been given to ways of stimulating changes in policy that will lead to the adoption of safer methods. More studies could be carried out of pesticide legislation in developing countries and of the problems encountered in the enforcement of existing regulations. Investigators have tended not to examine the implications of land tenure policies for health, apart from the effects of land distribution policies on the prevalence of specific diseases, such as malaria in the Amazon, and the health problems associated with large-scale transmigration. Much more could be done to assess the consequences for health of population migration associated with specific land tenure and rural development policies, and to find ways of preventing the adverse effects.

Research on health problems associated with industrial policies has focused on epidemiological studies of occupational diseases and accidents and has rarely explored the underlying causes of increases in ill-health. The researchers have tended to emphasize the need for adjustments in health policy—notably improvements in standard-setting, enforcement, occupational health services, and training, together with steps to ensure the availability of safety equipment—probably because there is some hope of action in these areas. To determine what changes are needed in overall strategies for industrial development is a far greater challenge. The literature on air and water pollution associated with industrialization in developing countries is still in its infancy. The lack of equipment for monitoring pollution, the inadequacy of the population data available, and the scarcity of studies on fundamental geographical differences affecting pollution concentrations have hindered research on the health effects of environmental pollution. In some major cities in developing countries, monitoring of the respiratory effects of industrial, energy, and vehicular air pollution has been increased. But the translation of such research into action is slow. Similarly, not enough attention has been paid to industrial policies that encourage the adoption of pollution-intensive technologies and the siting of industries in areas where the health risks from pollution may be greatest (owing to climate, population concentration, or other factors).

The situation with regard to studies on energy policies and health in developing countries is mixed. There is a growing literature on the relationship between domestic fuel use, respiratory infections, and low birth weight. Investigators have identified biofuel use as a major health hazard, but do not appear to be actively involved as yet in the development of practical policies and programmes to mitigate indoor air pollution either in rural or urban areas. In most countries, a careful assessment is needed of the effects on health of fuel-gathering requirements, changes in food preparation, or fuel substitution. Epidemiological evidence is gradually increasing on the links between energy use, outdoor levels of air pollution, and the incidence of respiratory problems, cancers, and stroke in the cities of the developing world. However, few studies have recommended specific regulatory measures for control of energy pollution. High-risk populations or districts have rarely been identified for targeting. Considerable attention has been paid to the effects of hydropower development projects on health, the primary risks are well-known, and health authorities are beginning to play a more important role in the design and implementation of these projects.

Some links between health and housing conditions have been well documented. However, in considering the health problems of urban slums and squatter settlements, investigators only rarely explore the broader aspects of housing policy, such as the effects of building restrictions, land tenure requirements, and the allocation of limited urban public services. The high cost of rented government housing and the excessive cost of the housing put up in sites-and-services projects have been linked to reduced spending on food by low-income urban populations, with potentially adverse effects on their nutritional status. Additional research is needed to ascertain the strength of this association, and to explore possible ways of avoiding deleterious trade-offs between expenditure on housing and expenditure on food in family budgets. Yet health authorities have not been actively engaged in the design or implementation of urban housing policies. In some areas, housing standards, based on outdated or inappropriate public health values, have proved difficult to implement, even counterproductive. On the whole, housing policy has paid little attention to disease control or public health programmes, and health services are often treated as secondary objectives in projects for infrastructure development.

Problems of implementation

Several problems have hindered the implementation of policy changes to mitigate the negative health impacts of macroeconomic policies. First, there has been the problem of uncertainty about the association. While it is now generally agreed that macroeconomic policies can affect health conditions among the poor in developing countries, debate continues on the degree or, in some cases, even the direction of their impact. Evidence from country studies is conflicting, and many effects may not be apparent in the short run. Methodological problems have contributed to this uncertainty, especially in attempts to determine the links between effects on nutrition and health conditions. Institutional and political biases have also obstructed implementation. Historically, national and international development agencies have concentrated on promoting economic growth, and have assumed that the resultant benefits would trickle down to the poor. Only recently have health components been introduced into adjustment programmes in recognition of the need to consider the distributional consequences of macroeconomic policy. Policy-makers increasingly agree about the need for measures to alleviate at least the short-term transitional costs of adjustment that fall, or are likely to fall (even if they cannot be measured with certainty), on the poor in developing countries. But, when implemented, these measures may not be appropriately targeted to the people most in need, and they are also likely to be rather more concerned with acute needs than with long-term health problems.

In agricultural policy as well, a mixture of technical, institutional, and political obstacles prevents the implementation of measures to improve health. Government agencies responsible for the development of irrigation systems are usually competing for limited resources with agencies responsible for other aspects of economic development. They may therefore be unwilling to assess potential negative effects on health (and the associated costs) during the planning of irrigation projects. Irrigation development policies have run into difficulties in focusing attention on safe methods for management and operation of these systems so as to reduce potential health risks. Measures aimed at land tenure reform (including land-titling projects, land redistribution and land grant programmes, and resettlement programmes) could have a positive impact on health. But they are likely to encounter serious political opposition from those whose economic interests are threatened. Most agricultural development projects involving population migration and resettlement now draw up plans to reduce health risks and meet the health needs of the populations involved. However, many authorities have been remiss in their implementation of such plans for political and economic reasons. With regard to pesticides, most governments in developing countries lack the financial, institutional, and human resources for the effective implementation of health and safety guidelines with regard to these hazardous chemicals. At present, many countries even lack the infrastructure to monitor the incidence and nature of cases of accidental poisoning by pesticides.

Efforts to mitigate the negative effects of industrial policies on health are also faced with numerous obstacles. Policies aimed at reducing pollution, the incidence of accidents, and associated health risks for workers or communities may conflict with national aims for industrial growth and be opposed by political interests accordingly. Pollution-prone industries and small-scale enterprises may expand more rapidly than the institutional capacity of a government to control the health and safety risks associated with industrialization. Efforts to improve occupational safety and health are impeded by various institutional obstacles: the overlapping of administrative responsibilities between health departments, industrial officials, and planners; the lack of arrangements for the registration and inspection of small-scale, informal, or rural enterprises; and the absence of coherent and implementable standards. The opposition of management, especially in countries with a strong private sector and weak labour organizations, can undercut government efforts to promote safety and health both inside and outside the factory. Pollution control measures may be too expensive or complicated for many companies in developing countries. In addition, for political reasons, government officials may fail to enforce pollution standards in the case of certain favoured firms, domestic or foreign. Some countries, however, are gradually adopting measures to control the negative social costs of industrial growth. These policies will need continued support to be sustainable.

Energy policies incorporating health considerations are only now developing. The absence of implementable energy policies in the past has contributed to fuel scarcity and fuel poverty, with profound repercussions on the health of poor rural and urban households. Energy programmes aimed at making wood fuel more accessible may conflict with others aimed at reducing reliance on unsafe fuels. More coordination and additional resources are required to widen the dissemination of safe and efficient technology. Programmes to improve cooking-stoves have often failed, because they do not promote technology that is affordable and amenable to the continuation of traditional cooking practices. Some advances have been made in improving the cultural acceptability of changes in cooking techniques, and more attention is being paid to the modernization of existing stoves. Such developments should, however, be accompanied by educational campaigns to ensure that the health benefits of fuel-efficient stoves are well understood. Fuel subsidies have often benefited moderate-income groups more than the low-income populations originally targeted, and many fuel subsidy programmes have been eliminated because of a shortage of government funds. Feasible means of achieving a significant reduction in pollution from industrial energy sources are still elusive. In the case of hydroelectric projects, improved guidelines exist on health assessment, safety, disease prevention, and population resettlement and rehabilitation. However, these guidelines may be applied only in large dam projects monitored by donor agencies. It is unclear whether countries will be prepared to respond to the long-term health consequences of the environmental disruption associated with such projects.

Problems in the implementation of housing policies may be due to limited resources, unattainable goals, institutional obstacles, and political pressures. Housing programmes designed to assist low-income populations may remove people from existing slums and squatter settlements with their own infrastructure, self-constructed shelter, and community services, and then fail to provide adequate resources for equal facilities in new housing developments—thereby creating new environmental health risks. Funding for housing programmes may include initial inputs of cash, credit, and resources, but then fail to provide adequately for the long-term development needs of the community. The financing procedures may be unduly complicated, making the resources inaccessible to many of the people targeted for assistance and reducing the potential for health improvements. Improper targeting of programmes can result in benefits being carried over to moderate-income groups, while the majority of low-income groups go without. Zoning and density regulations to protect areas of moderate-income housing and commercial properties may prevent the permanent settlement of populations or lead to their settlement in hazardous localities (industrial zones, inaccessible outlying areas, or areas with poor-quality soil). Lack of planning, financial resources, or administrative capability may prevent the development of health services and public health measures within housing programmes. Lack of coordination between housing, infrastructure, and health officials can also obstruct the effective implementation of the health components of housing programmes.

Exacerbation of poverty

A common theme runs throughout the above discussion: development policies can adversely affect health conditions, both directly (for example, through the proliferation of disease vectors or the introduction of toxic pollutants) and also indirectly—mainly by increasing household poverty. This suggests that a large group of adverse health conditions are basically the result of reductions in disposable income among the poor. At the extremes of poverty, most household income is spent on food and water (if the latter is not available free), plus a smaller amount on shelter, leaving little surplus. For the poor people concerned, reduced income leads to malnutrition and related health problems. Reduced income for the very poor can result from policies that cause either a reduction in income across the population or increased maldistribution of income. Both are likely to have an adverse effect on health conditions for the poor. Policies that increase the prices of necessary items, such as food, fuel, or housing, can have profound repercussions on health. If consumption is price-inelastic—i.e., a price increase will not lead to a decrease in consumption— then the policy will have the effect of reducing disposable income in other respects. If consumption is price-elastic, then the particular item will be used less, and health will be affected accordingly.

Development policy can thus have the unintended consequence of exacerbating poverty. Poverty can be made harsher in the preliminary phases of a development policy, as happens with economic stabilization and adjustment policies. Alternatively, increased poverty may be the long-term result of a policy. For example, a scheme for water resource development or an industrial project can lead to the dislocation of populations without adequate planning for resettlement, land provision, or job creation. The problems and the solutions here lie within the sphere of economic policy, and health changes are a consequence of economic policy. Epidemiologists may be able to estimate the health consequences of an anticipated level of poverty, but the economic issues are primary, and are where preventive action should be directed. This cluster of issues, in aggregate, is of critical importance for health.

Many of the problems encountered in relating broad development policies to health are thus specific examples of a more general problem. Those groups propounding a particular development policy usually have one primary aim in view. Other unintended effects, whether good or ill, tend to be viewed as secondary. Yet good policies need to be thought out fully in terms of their numerous short- and long-range effects. This has rarely been done where these effects are in the areas of the environment and health.

Two major research approaches will be required to deal adequately with the policy effects that impoverish households selectively. The first approach consists of economic analysis to determine how to protect the poor. The second is primarily epidemiological and seeks to determine the effects of increasing poverty on health under various circumstances. By breaking down these approaches, it is possible to reduce the need for complex interdisciplinary collaboration, simplify the list of tasks to be performed, and make it unnecessary to pass on the responsibility to other researchers or policy-makers.

Research needs

This review has demonstrated that the evaluation of development policies has not paid enough attention to their effects on health, that health research has tended not to examine development policies as immediate and underlying causes of ill-health, and that the improvement of health conditions is often hindered by the countless problems involved in the implementation of these policies. In addition, the absence of explicit policy can have adverse effects on health. Yet, in each sector, there are examples of how intersectoral research can successfully assess and address ensuing health problems. The successes recorded, however, are modest in scope compared with the problems still lacking attention.

A great many aspects of the relationship between development policy and health call for research. What should have priority? For example, ground-clearing exercises of limited scope could be carried out in areas where data are fragmentary and have not been brought together, or where more than one discipline is concerned and nobody has yet summarized the available information. These would involve a number of small, but useful tasks. To achieve a deeper understanding of the matter, a more thorough study of specific situations is required. For such studies to be of value, selection is essential.

Identifying and classifying gaps in research, as has been done in this review, could help to clarify the research agenda. This approach could be useful for avoiding complex questions that are unlikely to lead to satisfactory answers. Most of the important questions are difficult to pursue, and to get clear answers will be quite a costly business. It is therefore important to decide which are the important questions and to keep the list as short as possible.

A variety of factors have contributed to the large gaps that exist in our understanding of the relationship between development policies and health conditions. First there are practical and cultural factors specifically affecting research workers. Being multidisciplinary, this field of research is difficult to master in terms of the skills and disciplines required, and yet it is of low status, as involving neither purely economic policy nor purely health research. Economists and epidemiologists have different research expectations and habits. Hybrid studies of policy effects are likely to be frustrating to research workers, and the concept of rigour (so closely linked to scientific respectability) is very different in each of the disciplines involved.

Thus, if the research is to be performed successfully, key issues must be clarified as far as possible. Many steps are involved from policy formulation, through implementation, to health effects. The processes need to be sorted out and broken down as far as possible. Several economic policies may converge to affect disposable income, for example, and the latter in turn may influence health. Since only a few development policies can be the subject of pilot studies, the most important questions need to be identified at every stage in the path that leads from policy formulation to health effects, so that each of the processes involved can be studied in the most appropriate way.

Development policies may have a profound effect on health, but so broad and pervasive are such policies that the causal chain from policy to health effects is far from clear, and certainty about quantitative relationships is hard to come by. Activities in the implementation of a policy—programmes or specific projects—may be more tractable. It is therefore not surprising that the clearest understanding of the relationship between development policies and health problems exists in respect of discrete projects. These are more amenable to the methods of the field epidemiologist and the social scientist.

A number of research methodologies are suitable for assessing short- and long-term health effects of development policies. These include: risk measurement and assessment; analysis of social and environmental impact; cost-benefit analysis and cost-effectiveness studies; analysis of institutional policies and planning systems; controlled intervention studies; sociological and anthropological studies; large-project evaluation; and techniques for the assessment of macroeconomic policies. A discussion of the advantages and disadvantages of each of these approaches is beyond the scope of this review. However, for interdisciplinary work in this area to be well designed, implementable, and productive, such discussion must take place.

Researchers need to assess how complex interdisciplinary work can be carried out, and how problem areas can be identified. While research on whole systems will be imperative, a balance must be struck with research activities and policy modifications in the distinct but interlocking fields that are affected by the development policies discussed here. The main difficulties likely to be encountered will concern the rigour with which causality is demonstrated.

Extrapolation from the results of slow changes in policy or happenings in another period may be defective. A study of controlled policy measures will probably be the most instructive of any, both for understanding the links between development policy and health and for determining how best to improve matters.

It is clear from the preceding chapters that the effects of development policies on health are diverse, numerous, and often difficult to measure. Evidence from well-studied analogous topics (such as the relationship of improved water supply to health) suggests that to gain epidemiologically elegant and complete data is an elusive goal. If the policy consequences can be classified and arranged in some appropriate way, this may clarify and limit the relevant epidemiological consequences and also indicate what agencies should be responsible for further analysis and for solving outstanding problems. Once interventions are being considered, it becomes even more important to separate the processes involved. Interdisciplinary and intersectoral work is harder in practice. It is therefore necessary to have a clear picture of the components in a complex picture and to know exactly who is responsible for each aspect.

Case studies represent an important first step in pursuing and illuminating the questions raised in this review, and can be helpful in providing evidence of discrete causal relationships between development policies and health conditions in specific situations. In addition, they can identify some of the processes involved in the development, implementation, and evaluation of policies, and point to ways of assessing the costs and benefits of potential policy measures. The inclusion of measures that have successfully helped to reduce health risks, control disease, or provide needed health services would be particularly useful. On the basis of such case studies, more complex research questions could then be explored, and cross-national comparisons developed.

Ultimately, the purpose of research in the areas just outlined is both to advance our understanding of how best to use development policies in improving health conditions for poor populations in developing countries, and to stimulate the relevant action. However, a great problem faced by studies of this type is the difficulty of analysing complex interactions to produce operationally manageable conclusions. The research topic explored, the tools applied, and the resulting conclusions must therefore be well defined and relevant to policy-makers.

How policy analysts present their results can affect the willingness of decision-makers to take action and modify development policies. For policy-makers to respond effectively to an unintended